Family Support Programs and Rehabilitation

A Cognitive–Behavioral Approach to Traumatic Brain Injury

CRITICAL ISSUES IN NEUROPSYCHOLOGY

Series Editors

Antonio E. Puente
University of North Carolina, Wilmington

Cecil R. Reynolds
Texas A&M University

Current Volumes in this Series

BEHAVIORAL INTERVENTIONS WITH BRAIN-INJURED CHILDREN
A. MacNeill Horton, Jr.

CLINICAL NEUROPSYCHOLOGICAL ASSESSMENT:
A Cognitive Approach
Edited by Robert L. Mapou and Jack Spector

FAMILY SUPPORT PROGRAMS AND REHABILITATION:
A Cognitive–Behavioral Approach to Traumatic Brain Injury
Louise Margaret Smith and Hamish P. D. Godfrey

NEUROPSYCHOLOGICAL EVALUATION OF THE
SPANISH SPEAKER
Alfredo Ardila, Monica Rosselli, and Antonio E. Puente

NEUROPSYCHOLOGICAL EXPLORATIONS OF
MEMORY AND COGNITION:
Essays in Honor of Nelson Butters
Edited by Laird S. Cermak

NEUROPSYCHOLOGICAL TOXICOLOGY:
Identification and Assessment of Human Neurotoxic Syndromes,
Second Edition
David E. Hartman

THE NEUROPSYCHOLOGY OF ATTENTION
Ronald A. Cohen

A PRACTICAL GUIDE TO HEAD INJURY REHABILITATION:
A Focus on Postacute Residential Treatment
Michael D. Wesolowski and Arnie H. Zencius

PRACTITIONER'S GUIDE TO CLINICAL NEUROPSYCHOLOGY
Robert M. Anderson, Jr.

A Continuation Order Plan is available for this series. A continuation order will bring delivery of each new volume immediately upon publication. Volumes are billed only upon actual shipment. For further information please contact the publisher.

Family Support Programs and Rehabilitation

A Cognitive–Behavioral Approach to Traumatic Brain Injury

Louise Margaret Smith and
Hamish P. D. Godfrey
University of Otago
Dunedin, New Zealand

Springer Science+Business Media, LLC

Library of Congress Cataloging-in-Publication Data

On file

ISBN 978-1-4899-0238-2 ISBN 978-1-4899-0236-8 (eBook)
DOI 10.1007/978-1-4899-0236-8

Originally published by Plenum Press, New York in 1995
Softcover reprint of the hardcover 1st edition 1995

10 9 8 7 6 5 4 3 2 1

Foreword

The permanent effects of traumatic brain injury (TBI) are not limited to the person who suffers the injury. People who care for the individual, particularly family members, suffer in various ways. Family members are often confused as to the behavioral and neuropsychological changes that they see in a brain-injured relative. They can become frustrated and angry when the individual does not return to premorbid levels of functioning. They can become tired and worn down from repeated problems in trying to manage the individual's difficulties while having only fragmented information regarding them.

Drs. Smith and Godfrey have provided a useful service for family members by summarizing important neuropsychological changes associated with TBI and providing practical guidelines for coping with these problems.

While the neuropsychological problems they describe are not completely understood, the authors provide a useful description of many of the neurobehavioral problems seen following TBI in young adults. They attempt to provide guidelines for family members that have practical utility in understanding and managing these patients. Theirs is a cognitive–behavioral approach that can have utility for this group of individuals. I applaud their efforts to provide something systematic and practical for family members.

The research findings they report in this volume highlight the fact that if family members are given information and support, their emotional distress may not worsen with time. The opposite pattern, however, is frequently seen when family members are not given help. The family's distress level, as well as the patient's, can increase with time without appropriate professional help.

This book is useful because it provides families with some understanding of the many problems associated with TBI. It also attempts to provide guidelines to help patients manage many of these problems. Family members should be warned, however, that they as well as therapists do not have a simple "cookbook" for solving the serious problems of TBI individuals. In fact, there are very few cures for any of these behavioral problems. With appropriate knowledge about the patients and appropriate ways of knowing how to approach them, however, many of the problems can be managed more effectively. The research findings reported by Smith and Godfrey provide indirect evidence for this point of view.

An extremely important and difficult issue in working with patients who have suffered TBI is the problem of altered self-awareness or posttraumatic insight disorder, as Dr. Godfrey refers to it. This problem is indeed complicated and one that requires further empirical evaluation. If families are aware of the complexities of this problem and the need to understand it, they will be able to better manage the individuals who suffer these devastating injuries.

Smith and Godfrey's book is a welcome addition to our body of knowledge that can be passed on to family members in an effort to assist them in coping with a loved one who has suffered traumatic injury to the brain.

GEORGE P. PRIGATANO
Barrow Neurological Institute
Phoenix, Arizona

Preface

During the past decade, there has been a wealth of new research on the psychosocial effects of traumatic brain injury (TBI). This research boom reflects a growing recognition that psychosocial problems represent the greatest difficulty for individuals affected by TBI. The majority of TBI individuals return home after acute medical treatment. Consequently, families are the primary long-term caregivers for individuals affected by TBI. With recognition of this state of affairs, an important objective of research on the psychosocial effects of TBI has been to more fully understand how families respond to the challenge of living with a relative who has suffered a TBI.

Unfortunately, families are often provided with limited information, support, or practical advice about how to cope with the demands of living with a TBI relative. These demands are primarily psychosocial in nature, and they reflect difficulties in understanding and coping with a TBI relative who may now display adverse personality changes and cognitive impairment. Not surprisingly, research has convincingly documented a pattern of increasing burden for such families, tending to worsen with increasing time after the TBI relative returns to the home environment. To date, there has been very little, if any, evaluation of programs designed to prevent or ameliorate the burden on families affected by TBI.

The primary aim of this volume is to encourage practitioners working with TBI individuals to address psychosocial problems and to do so within the family context. The book is intended for a wide audience, including clinical neuropsychologists, clinical psychologists, nurses, occupational therapists, neurologists, psychiatrists, and medical students, as well as the families who are directly affected by TBI. Two features have been employed to facilitate the reader's use of the intervention strategies described. First, we have made extensive use of procedural summaries in which intervention strategies are described in detailed, easy-to-follow steps. Second, we have included numerous case descriptions to illustrate the application of intervention techniques.

Traumatic brain injury often results in a complex array of adverse psychosocial effects. In Chapter 1, an overview of these effects is provided, followed by a review of rehabilitation research in Chapter 2. Chapters 3 through 6 describe the family support programs, including intervention strategies designed to compensate for cognitive impairment, enhance emotional adjustment, improve social competency, and foster family adaptation. A secondary aim of this volume is to present the results of a controlled evaluation of the family support program. These results are presented in Chapter 7, in which the efficacy of the family support program is compared with that of hospital-based care. Finally, the study findings and their wider clinical implications are discussed in Chapter 8.

We are greatly indebted to many individuals who assisted in this study and the earlier research on which it was partly based. First, we thank the families who willingly participated in the research program over a lengthy time period. Second, the University of Otago provided funding without which this study would not have been possible. In particular, we are very grateful to Professor Geoffrey White, Head of the Psychology Department, for his practical support and advice. Third, we greatly appreciate the support we have received from colleagues. We have benefited greatly from working with Barry Longmore, an outstanding clinician who served as clinical supervisor during one year of the study. Samir Bishara provided medical assessments of study participants and has been a supportive colleague and research collaborator for many years. Robert Knight has been a helpful advisor and offered good-humored support during this and earlier research. Thanks also to Isabel Campbell for her skillful typing of the manuscript.

Finally, we dedicate this book to our parents, who supported us for such a long time and provided us with an understanding of the importance of family.

Contents

1

Psychosocial Effects of Traumatic Brain Injury

INTRODUCTION

More than 50,000 people suffer traumatic brain injury (TBI) in the United States each year (Kirn, 1987). The size of the population affected by TBI is alarming when one considers that this number increases cumulatively across time (Volpe & McDowell, 1990) and that survival rates are also increasing due to medical advances (Christensen, Pinner, Moller Pedersen, Teasdale, & Trexler, 1992). Unfortunately, the majority of TBI individuals are left with permanent and adverse personality change and cognitive impairment (Lezak, 1978). As a consequence of these changes, persons who sustain TBI often are unable to maintain their preinjury social roles (Oddy, Humphrey, & Uttley, 1978b) and experience reactive emotional problems (Godfrey, Partridge, Knight, & Bishara, 1993b). The vast majority of TBI patients are discharged home after hospitalization (Liss & Willer, 1990), and their families serve as primary caregivers (Brooks, 1991). Not surprisingly, many families experience chronic burden, which tends to worsen with the increasing time after injury (Livingston, Brooks, & Bond, 1985a).

This book describes a family-based approach to rehabilitation following TBI that we have called the *family support program*. By way of background, Chapters 1 and 2 include a brief review of research on the long-term psychosocial effects of TBI and the rehabilitation approaches that have been utilized in an attempt to ameliorate these effects. Chapters 3 through 6 describe the family support program in detail, along with the results of single case studies. Chapters 7 and 8 present the results of a controlled evaluation of the family support program and discuss the implications of these results. In this chapter, the review of research findings is restricted to studies of individuals who have sustained moderate to severe TBI and who have been discharged from the hospital in a conscious state. Moderate to severe TBI has been defined by Glasgow Coma Scale (Jennett &

Teasdale, 1981) scores of 3–12 on hospital admission (Prigatano, 1992), or by posttraumatic amnesia lasting more than 24 hours (W. R. Russell, 1971), or by both criteria.

PHYSICAL EFFECTS

Traumatic brain injury refers to damage that results from blunt trauma in which the skull is not pierced (Partridge, 1991). Although it is often referred to as "closed head injury," the term "traumatic brain injury" is preferable because it emphasizes that the brain has been damaged secondary to external forces (Prigatano, 1992). TBI is generally associated with car accidents, falls, or sporting accidents (Bishara, Partridge, Godfrey, & Knight, 1992; Frankowski, 1986). Two primary types of damage usually occur: diffuse axonal shearing and focal cerebral contusions (Benedict, 1989). Diffuse axonal shearing is a consequence of the rotational forces that occur during acceleration or deceleration at the time of impact (Rose, 1988; W. R. Russell, 1971). Centripetal and centrifugal forces produce widespread axonal shearing (Meier, Strauman, & Thompson, 1987), particularly in the parasagittal white matter (Benedict, 1989). This diffuse damage is particularly significant in that it is thought to result in more serious functional impairment than is caused by localized injury (Molloy, 1983).

Focal cerebral contusions normally occur as a consequence of the rotational movements of the frontal and temporal lobes against the bony ridges in the corresponding inside area of the skull. "Coup" contusions occur at the site of injury, while "contracoup" contusions are diametrically opposite and are caused by changes in intracranial pressure (Richardson, 1990). Secondary damage may also occur in the form of hematomas, cerebral edema, increased intracranial pressure, ischemic brain damage, and posttraumatic epilepsy. The actual configuration of neuropathology will differ greatly from patient to patient (Gordon & Hibbard, 1992). Consequently, the effects of TBI also vary greatly from individual to individual, and it is this heterogeneity of effect that complicates research on psychosocial outcome after TBI (Adamovich, Henderson, & Auerbach, 1985).

Neurophysical disability is the most conspicuous form of residual impairment following TBI (Richardson, 1990), and historically this aspect of functioning was the focus of much early research (e.g., Symonds, 1962). A wide range of neurophysical disabilities may result from TBI, including visual difficulties, language impairment, sensorimotor deficits, hemiparesis (Zahara & Cuvo, 1984), nutritional deficits (Brooke et al., 1989), ataxia, facial palsies, anosmia, and posttraumatic epilepsy (Jennett & Teasdale, 1981). It is estimated that about 40% of TBI patients suffer some form of clinically significant neurophysical disability (Perry, 1983), which will tend to resolve during the first few months after injury

(Jennett & Teasdale, 1981). However, a minority of TBI patients experience chronic neurophysical difficulties that have been documented as long as 10–15 years after injury (Thomsen, 1984), suggesting that for some TBI patients, neurophysical disability is permanent. The research interest in neurophysical disabilities has waned over the past decade as it has become increasingly apparent that the long-term psychosocial sequelae exceed the physical sequelae as the primary cause of concern for both the patients and their families (Ben-Yishay et al., 1985; Brooks, 1984; Panting & Merry, 1972; Soderstrom, Fogelsjoo, & Fugl-Meyer, 1988; Tate, 1987a).

COGNITIVE IMPAIRMENT

Few people who sustain severe traumatic head injury escape without some degree of chronic cognitive impairment. For example, Tate, Fenelon, Manning, and Hunter (1991) found that 70% of a consecutive series of 100 TBI patients were left with cognitive impairment as late as 6 years after injury. Interest in the area of cognitive impairment after TBI has burgeoned in the last two decades. It is now hypothesized to be the core deficit underlying a wide variety of long-term psychosocial effects, including behavioral disturbance (Malec, 1984), communication disorders (Malkmus, 1989), poor vocational adjustment (Cancelliere, Moncada, & Reid, 1991), and lack of awareness of disability (Klonoff, O'Brien, Prigatano, Chiapello, & Cunningham, 1989). Cognitive impairment is thought to encompass perception, processing of abstract information, executive functioning (i.e., planning, self-monitoring, goal setting), learning, attention, speed of information processing, language, and memory (Molloy, 1983; Szekeres, Ylvisaker, & Cohen, 1987; Zahara & Cuvo, 1984). These deficits present a significant obstacle to adjustment after TBI, in that they can impede rehabilitation efforts (Cicerone & Wood, 1987; Richardson, 1990; Series, 1992). In the following section, research on each of these areas of cognitive impairment is briefly summarized.

Intellectual Functioning

Intellectual impairment is relatively common following TBI (McClelland, 1988), with IQ scores decrementing approximately 15 points on average (e.g., Becker, 1975). Impairment of intellect tends to be greatest on performance tasks (e.g., Dye, Saxon, & Milby, 1981), with verbal intelligence remaining relatively spared (Mandelberg & Brooks, 1975). The extent to which intellectual functioning recovers remains controversial, in part because of difficulty in distinguishing improvement due to practice from genuine recovery (for a discussion on this issue, see Richardson, 1990, pp. 154–157).

Memory

Memory impairment is the most common type of cognitive deficit found on neuropsychological testing (Tate et al., 1991) and identified by relatives (Oddy, Coughlan, Tyerman, & Jenkins, 1985) following TBI. Memory impairment tends to be chronic in nature and is often evident several years following injury. Estimates of the risk of chronic memory impairment following TBI are typically between 50% and 70% (Brooks, 1984; Brooks, Campsie, Symington, Beattie, & McKinlay, 1986; McKinlay, Brooks, Bond, Martinage, & Marshall, 1981). This high risk of memory impairment in part reflects the vulnerability of the temporal lobes to localized damage at the time of injury (Cancelliere et al., 1991) and the high probability of ischemic damage to the hippocampal regions following TBI (Prigatano & Fordyce, 1986a).

Memory is not only very commonly impaired following head injury, but also disproportionately impaired relative to intellectual functioning (Levin, Goldstein, High, & Eisenberg, 1988). This finding suggests that memory impairment is not part of a global impairment of cognitive ability, but rather a relatively specific cognitive impairment. Memory impairment following TBI shares many of the features of dysmnesia resulting from other etiologies (Levin, 1990b). Thus, TBI patients' poor performance on commonly used verbal learning tests such as the Selective Reminding Test (Marsh, Knight, & Godfrey, 1990; Paniak, Shore, & Rourke, 1989) and the California Verbal Learning Test (Crosson, Novack, Trenerry, & Craig, 1988) reflect disrupted memory processes such as selective retrieval (e.g., Vakil, Arbell, Gozlan, Hoofien, & Blachstein, 1992). However, many aspects of learning and remembering, such as semantic memory processes, are relatively unimpaired following TBI (F. C. Goldstein, Levin, & Boake, 1989; Levin & Goldstein, 1986; Schmitter-Edgecombe, Marks, & Fahy, 1993).

TBI patients' performance on memory tests does improve over the first year following injury (Brooks & Aughton, 1979). However, the rate of recovery thereafter tends to be variable, and the majority of TBI patients are left with some degree of residual memory impairment (Tate et al., 1991). The clinical significance of memory impairments has been validated by the reports of TBI patients' relatives (Brooks et al., 1986) and by the finding of an association between severity of memory impairment and failure to return to work after injury (Brooks, McKinlay, Symington, Beattie, & Campsie, 1987; Godfrey, Bishara, Partridge, & Knight, 1993a).

Information-Processing Speed

TBI individuals perform more slowly on a wide range of mental tasks (Berrol, 1990). Furthermore, their performance becomes disproportionately worse as the task demands increase (Van Zomeren, Brouwer, & Deelman, 1984). Slowing of performance is thought to occur almost universally after TBI (Ponsford & Kinsella, 1988) and can be readily documented on clinical tests such as the Paced Auditory Serial-Addition Task (Gronwall, 1977). Performance slowing is thought to reflect disruption of mediobasal frontal and medial temporal structures (Webster & Scott, 1983). Although impairment of speed of information processing may lessen in severity over the course of recovery, significant residual impairment is often evident many months or years postinjury (Sohlberg & Mateer, 1987).

Research on mental slowing following TBI has largely been conducted within an information-processing experimental paradigm (Broadbent, 1958) that owes much to analogies with computer processing. The classic experimental task for documenting slowed performance following TBI is choice reaction time (e.g., Van Zomeren & Deelman, 1976). TBI individuals' poorer performance on tasks such as these is thought to reflect primarily a slowing of information processing rather than, for example, an impairment of selective attention (Ponsford & Kinsella, 1992). Slowing of information processing is thought to underlie a wide range of other cognitive impairments following TBI (Richardson, 1990), including memory deficit (Haut, Petros, Frank, & Haut, 1991), problem-solving difficulties, and impaired communication (Barry & Riley, 1987; Ponsford & Kinsella, 1988). A number of recent studies have attempted to determine the stage of information processing most affected after TBI. These studies have documented problems with both stimulus encoding and response selection (Schmitter-Edgecombe, Marks, Fahey, & Long, 1992; Shum, McFarland, Bain, & Humphreys, 1990).

Executive Functioning

The effect of TBI on executive functioning (Stuss & Benson, 1984) has received much less research consideration than either memory impairment or slowing of information processing, even though executive dysfunction is a common sequela of TBI (Stuss & Gow, 1992). Executive dysfunction following TBI is thought to involve many cognitive abilities and includes the following: a lack of response initiation and generation (Crowe, 1992), difficulty in planning goal-directed behavior (Vilkki, 1992), disorders of judgment and reasoning (F. C. Goldstein & Levin, 1991), inability to self-regulate, and inflexibility of thinking (F. C. Goldstein & Levin, 1987; Lezak, 1987; Prigatano & Fordyce, 1986a; Ylvisaker & Szekeres, 1989). There have been relatively few empirical studies in this area, and research to date has been hampered by the imprecise definition of executive functioning. Perhaps not surprisingly, strategies for ameliorating executive dysfunction are not well developed. Burke, Zencius, Wesolowski, and Doubleday (1991) rightly comment that executive-function disorders remain an enigma.

Language

Clinical aphasia is relatively rare following TBI. For example, Heilman, Safran, and Geschwin (1971) reported only 13 definite cases of aphasia in a sample of 750 consecutive hospital admissions for TBI. However, milder forms of expressive and receptive language disturbance are common following TBI (Sarno, 1988). These language deficits are evidenced by poorer performance on measures such as the Token Test and verbal fluency tasks and have been termed "subclinical aphasia" (Sarno, 1980). Language disturbance is also apparent in the subtly degraded speech evidenced by many TBI patients. Recent studies employing discourse analysis have documented impoverished cohesion, syntax, productivity, content, and clarity of language use in speech following TBI (Glosser & Deser, 1990; Liles, Coelho, Duffy, & Zalagens, 1989; Mentis & Prutting, 1987).

Although the degree of language impairment following TBI is often relatively mild, recent findings suggest that even mild impairment of language may be clinically significant. For example, observational studies have found that impoverished speech content is associated with the affected individuals' being perceived as socially unrewarding (Godfrey, Knight, Marsh, Moroney, & Bishara, 1989). Apparently, mild language disturbance following TBI has significant social consequences, as inability to make a positive social impression is one mechanism by which TBI individuals become socially isolated (Spence, Godfrey, Bishara, & Knight, 1993; Tate, Lulham, Broe, Strettles, & Pfaff, 1989). Furthermore, family members, who often serve as the TBI individual's primary social support (Elsass & Kinsella, 1987), may experience significant burden in attempting to maintain verbal interactions with a socially unresponsive TBI individual who requires considerable prompting (Godfrey, Knight, & Bishara, 1991).

PERSONALITY CHANGE

Family members often comment that the TBI individual "is not the same person he was before the injury." In making such observations, family members are referring to the personality change (Prigatano, 1992) they have observed in their TBI relative. In its milder form, personality change impairs the TBI victim's interpersonal competency so subtly that it may not be obvious to the naïve observer. This impairment may be characterized by a range of pathological features, including the following: impoverished verbal fluency (Brooks & Aughton, 1979), inability to utilize environmental cues (Giles & Clark-Wilson, 1988a, b), use of inappropriate speech forms and gestures, expansive talk (Giles, Fussey, & Burgess, 1988), impaired social perceptiveness (Lezak, 1978), tangentiality (Prigatano, Roueche, & Fordyce, 1986b), failure to initiate and maintain conversation, poor eye contact, negative affective content in speech (Brotherton, Thomas,

Wisotzek, & Milan, 1988), difficulty paying attention to what is said, and inability to express thoughts accurately (Richardson, 1990).

Subtle impairment of interpersonal competency is a central hallmark of TBI sequelae. For example, Lezak (1987) followed up a group of TBI individuals from 1 month to 5 years postinjury and found that 90% reported difficulties with social interaction. Spence et al. (1993) found that over half their sample of TBI individuals were classified by clinical raters as socially unskilled (compared with 15% of orthopedic control subjects), suggesting that for many TBI individuals, impairment of interpersonal competency is of clinical severity.

For many TBI individuals, personality change may take a more obvious form that is characterized by an apparent reduction in motivation or lack of emotional control or both. Frequently cited personality changes of this type include increased childishness, irritability, anger (Lezak, 1987), and suspiciousness (Hinkeldey & Corrigan, 1990), on one hand, and aspontaneity (Thomsen, 1984) or lack of drive and initiative (Jennett & Teasdale, 1981), on the other. Personality changes involving reduced motivation or poor emotional control or both are common and tend to persist for years after injury. For example, 85% of relatives in one study reported that personality change had occurred (Thomsen, 1974), and these changes remained evident in 65% of these cases even 10–15 years postaccident (Thomsen, 1984). Similar discouraging results have been reported in many other studies (e.g., Brooks & McKinlay, 1983; Hinkeldey & Corrigan, 1990; Weddell, Oddy, & Jenkins, 1980).

In its most severe form, personality change following TBI has been referred to as a behavioral disorder (Tate, 1987b; Wood, 1988b). Behavioral disorders are usually classified as either behavioral excesses or deficits. Examples of behavioral excesses include impulsiveness, demanding behavior (Prigatano, 1987a), impatience, and verbal aggression (Goodman-Smith & Turnbull, 1983). Behavioral deficits commonly cited include a severe overall lack of drive, loss of motivation, apathy (Gloag, 1985), and lack of self-care skills (Zahara & Cuvo, 1984). Behavioral disorders are less common than milder forms of personality disorder, yet are nonetheless quite frequent (Burke, Wesolowski, & Guth, 1988a; Eames & Wood, 1985). When present, behavioral disorder has a profound and lasting effect upon TBI individuals and those around them (Brooks, 1988) and presents a formidable barrier to TBI individuals' resuming their preinjury social and vocational roles (Zahara & Cuvo, 1984; Haffey & Scibak, 1989).

The etiology of personality change following TBI is likely to be multifactorial (Prigatano, 1992). Neurological factors (e.g., Marquardt, Stoll, & Sussman, 1988) are possibly the largest single contributor to personality change; however, other factors such as psychological reactions (Prigatano & Fordyce, 1986a; Spence et al., 1993; Wood & Burgess, 1988), premorbid characteristics (Cicerone, 1989), level of adaptive coping responses, and extrinsic environmental factors (O'Shanick, 1989) are also likely to play an important role. Given that personality change is the most common symptom of TBI (Jennett & Teasdale, 1981) and the symptom that causes the greatest distress to families affected by TBI (Brooks & McKinlay, 1983), the paucity of research findings on this topic is regrettable.

SOCIAL ROLE FUNCTIONING

It has been suggested by many authors that most of the spontaneous recovery of abilities after TBI occurs within the first 6 months postinjury (e.g., Meier et al., 1987), with little change thereafter. However, it is now recognized that recovery proceeds well beyond the first few months or years (Cope, 1985; Cope, Cole, Hall, & Barkan, 1991a). Recovery of function is characterized by immense individual variability in terms of the nature and severity of impairments the TBI person is left with (Zahara & Cuvo, 1984). This variability is thought to be related to the type and severity of actual brain pathology, the use of alternative or redundant neural pathways (Jennett & Teasdale, 1981), the individual's coping ability (Prigatano, 1987b), and the extent to which residual abilities are used (Kalat, 1981).

Complete recovery is rare, however, and in general TBI results in long-standing cognitive and behavioral impairment (Christensen et al., 1992; Lezak, 1987). This is the case even when TBI patients have made a "good recovery" in medical terms (e.g., Bishara et al., 1992; Godfrey et al., 1993b). Unfortunately, these chronic cognitive and behavioral impairments have a profound impact on the TBI individual's ability to perform premorbid social roles. The following sections examine the long-term effects of TBI on social role functioning.

Vocational Adjustment

For many years, return to work has been utilized as the primary measure of social adjustment following TBI. The importance of returning to work stems largely from the role employment plays in maintaining the TBI individual's financial status and self-esteem (Wehman, Kreutzer, Stonnington, & Wood, 1988). There are dramatically different reports of rates of employment of TBI individuals following injury, ranging from as low as 7.5% (Thomsen, 1984) to as high as 82% (Oddy et al., 1978b). These differences are due largely to variations in sample characteristics (for a review of findings, see Kreutzer, Wehman, Morton, & Stonnington, 1991; Rao et al., 1990), with more severely injured victims being less likely to return to work (Stambrook, Moore, Peters, Deviaene, & Hawryluk, 1990). Reduced employability and lower vocational status are common problems following TBI and may reflect TBI individuals' tardiness, inappropriate verbal and sexual behavior, poor performance on work tasks, aggression, and poor initiation skills (Wehman et al., 1989a). As Lyons and Morse (1988) rightly comment, such behavior may be understood by therapists, but it is not often tolerated by employers or co-workers.

Factors that affect return to work are numerous. The strongest predictors are severity of injury and degree of neuropsychological impairment (Godfrey et al., 1993a; Kreutzer et al., 1991; Stambrook et al., 1990). However, education, age at injury (Jellinek & Harvey, 1982), communication disorders, cognitive and behavioral problems (Najenson, Groswasser, Mendelson, & Hackett, 1980), emotional control problems (Haffey & Lewis, 1989), alcohol abuse, failure to accept limitations, financial disincentives (Ben-Yishay, Silver, Piasetsky, & Rattok, 1987b), and personality change (Weddell et al., 1980) have also been implicated in failure to return to work.

Nonvocational Adjustment

The majority of people with TBI encounter difficulty in maintaining preinjury friendships and establishing new relationships (Lezak, 1987; Malkmus, 1989; Tate et al., 1989; Thomsen, 1984). For some TBI individuals, social isolation may be part of a depressive syndrome, but isolation may also occur in the absence of depression (Prigatano, 1987a). Clinically, it appears that after repeated failures in coping in social situations, TBI individuals simply avoid social situations. This avoidance is perilous in that it removes the person from social support, which serves as a buffer, reducing the impact of stress (Wagner, Williams, & Long, 1990). The results of research in this area are ominous. Lezak (1987) reports that at 5 years after injury, 90% of her sample experienced difficulties, with low levels of social contact. Two thirds of those in the study by Thomsen (1984) had no social contact beyond close family 10–15 years after injury. Controlled studies reveal similar findings, with TBI individuals receiving fewer visits, going on fewer social outings, dating less frequently, and relying more on family as a primary source of close attachment (Elsass & Kinsella, 1987; Oddy & Humphrey, 1980; Oddy et al., 1978b; Wagner et al., 1990; Weddell et al., 1980). Surprisingly, while TBI individuals do report a reduction in the extent of their social network following injury, they do not always report being dissatisfied with their social relationships (e.g., Elsass & Kinsella, 1987).

Leisure and recreational pursuits also appear to diminish following TBI (Tate et al., 1989; Thomsen, 1984). For example, Oddy et al. (1978b) found that TBI individuals reported significantly fewer leisure activities as compared to preinjury. In this study, 50% of the TBI individuals still engaged in fewer leisure activities at 1–2 years postaccident (Oddy & Humphrey, 1980). Weddell et al. (1980) replicated these results and noted continuing "social problems" at a 7-year follow-up (Oddy et al., 1985). Given that involvement in social and leisure pursuits is often minimal following TBI, it is not surprising that reports of loneliness and boredom are also common (e.g., Oddy et al., 1978b; Lezak, 1987; Thomsen, 1987).

EMOTIONAL ADJUSTMENT

Depression, catastrophic reactions (K. Goldstein, 1952), anxiety, and low self-esteem commonly occur following TBI (e.g., Fordyce, Roueche, & Prigatano, 1983; Lezak, 1987). For example, anxiety represents a chronic problem for one quarter to one half of TBI individuals (Lezak, 1987; Kinsella, Moran, Ford, & Ponsford, 1988; McKinlay et al., 1981; Tyerman & Humphrey, 1984). Similarly, rates of clinical depression in the TBI population have been estimated as being between 27% and 60% (Brooks et al., 1986; Elsass & Kinsella, 1987; Kinsella et al., 1988; Tyerman & Humphrey, 1984).

In the first few months after injury, however, TBI victims report low levels of anxiety and depression, which then increase to a peak at around 9–14 months (Fordyce et al., 1983; Lezak, 1987). This finding has led to suggestions that "denial" or "lack of awareness" is the primary emotional reaction in the first 6 months following injury (Cicerone, 1989). Godfrey et al. (1993b) have provided empirical evidence in support of this suggestion by documenting a positive relationship between TBI individuals' awareness of symptoms and their level of emotional dysfunction at different intervals from 6 months to 2 years after injury. They refer to the transient period of lack of awareness commonly evidenced shortly after injury as *posttraumatic insight disorder*. Insight disorder is a difficult construct to measure, but is a feature of TBI sequelae that is almost universally recognized by clinicians and researchers.

The etiology of insight disorder is poorly understood, but is thought to reflect disturbed neurophysiology (Slagle, 1990), neuropsychological impairment (Prigatano, 1987a), reactions to disability (Letoff, 1983; McClelland, 1988), or premorbid characterological problems (Prigatano, 1986). Currently, premorbid and reactive factors are stressed as etiological factors (Zahara & Cuvo, 1984), due to the lack of a strong relationship between actual brain damage and severity of emotional dysfunction (Prigatano, 1987a). McGlynn and Schacter (1990) provide an excellent overview of research on this topic.

Reports of psychosis after TBI are uncommon. Thomsen (1974) noted 8 cases of posttraumatic psychosis among 40 individuals with very severe TBI, and Lezak (1987) stated that 12–45% of her sample displayed some symptoms of hallucinatory and delusional ideation during a 5-year follow-up period. Psychopathology checklists such as the Brief Symptom Inventory have been employed in an attempt to determine the frequency of psychiatric disturbance following TBI, but these studies have tended to produce equivocal results. For example, Marsh et al. (1990) found no significant differences between TBI individuals and controls on the Symptom Distress Checklist 90, while Hinkeldey and Corrigan (1990) reported elevated paranoid ideation and psychoticism on a short form of the same measure. Further research is necessary to clarify the prevalence rates of psychotic symptoms following TBI. When psychotic symptoms are present, they are thought to be associated with localized damage to the limbic region and the frontal and temporal lobes (Slagle, 1990) or to reflect preexisting psychopathology (Prigatano, 1987a).

FAMILY ADJUSTMENT

In 1988, Muriel Lezak (1988) wrote a seminal paper entitled "Brain Damage Is a Family Affair." This title is indicative of the increasing acknowledgment of the impact that TBI has upon the whole family (Florian, Katz, & Lahav, 1991). The stresses families face after TBI are immense. Personality change is an ongoing source of strain (Hegeman, 1988; Klonoff & Prigatano, 1987). Failure to return to work results in loss of income (Rogers & Kreutzer, 1984; Liss & Willer, 1990), which is further compounded by medical bills and rehabilitation expenses. The role changes that occur following TBI make family restructuring unavoidable, and adjustment to this restructuring is often difficult (Zeigler, 1987; Mauss-Clum & Ryan, 1981). In addition, families carry primary responsibility for the postacute care of TBI individuals (Brooks, 1991), as over 80% of TBI patients return home on discharge (Liss & Willer, 1990). This can lead to social isolation (Rogers & Kreutzer, 1984), at the very time when the family is mourning the loss of a member who has not actually died (Zeigler, 1987). The psychological consequence of these stressors is elevated levels of depression (Lezak, 1978; Oddy, Humphrey, & Uttley, 1978a; Shaw & McMahon, 1990), anxiety (Livingston, Brooks, & Bond, 1985a,b), denial (Thomsen, 1984), anger (Lezak, 1987), guilt (Thomsen, 1974), sleeplessness (Panting & Merry, 1972), and stress and burden on family members (Florian et al., 1991; McKinlay et al., 1981).

Regrettably, family burden tends to worsen over time. For example, Livingston, Brooks, and Bond (1985a,b) found that female relatives of 42 TBI individuals reported gradually increasing levels of mood disturbance and decreasing marital and social adjustment during the first year after TBI. At the 1-year assessment, 30% of relatives were classified as clinically maladjusted on the General Health Questionnaire and 40% on the Leeds Anxiety Scale. As noted, family burden continues to increase over time, and severe burden has been documented as late as 7 years after injury by these researchers (Brooks et al., 1987a). Not surprisingly, family burden is associated with adverse changes in the TBI person's functioning (Brooks & McKinlay, 1983).

Relationships with partners appear to be particularly vulnerable following TBI. Half the wives in one survey endorsed the statement, "I'm married but I don't really have a husband" (Mauss-Clum & Ryan, 1981). Affectional and sexual needs are less often met, and the partner may struggle with loneliness (Lezak, 1978). Due to the lack of research in this area, it is not yet clear whether there is a higher divorce rate in couples affected by TBI. However, L. C. Peters, Stambrook, Moore, and Esses (1990) found that wives of severely injured TBI individuals perceive significantly greater marital dysfunction in the areas of affectional expression, dyadic consensus, and overall adjustment as compared with wives of men with minor and moderate head injuries and compared with wives of individuals with a spinal cord injury. It has been suggested that younger women tend to terminate relationships, while older women remain in relationships but operate in purely caretaker roles (Liss & Willer, 1990; Zeigler, 1987). Relationship difficulties can be intensified if the injured person's parents try to protect the TBI individual from divorce (Mauss-Clum & Ryan, 1981) or if the TBI individual competes with the children for attention and love from the noninjured partner (Florian et al., 1991).

CONCLUSIONS

To the casual observer, a TBI person may appear and behave the same way following injury (Gordon & Hibbard, 1992). Yet the research summarized in this chapter indicates that for many TBI individuals and their families, life will never again be the same. A high proportion of TBI individuals experience significant cognitive impairment, in particular impoverished memory and attentional abilities. Others display adverse personality changes such as impaired motivation and poor emotional control. Readjustment to the social world of friendships, leisure pursuits, and employment proves difficult in the face of reduced cognitive and interpersonal competency. These problems tend to be chronic, lasting many years after injury. In response to these problems, emotional reactions of anxiety and depression are common. Indeed, both TBI individuals and their families face immense changes as they struggle to readjust to life after traumatic brain injury.

2

Approaches to Rehabilitation Following Traumatic Brain Injury

Early approaches to traumatic brain injury (TBI) rehabilitation emphasized conservative management and the treatment of physical disability (Symonds, 1962). With increasing acknowledgment of the cognitive and behavioral sequelae of TBI, rehabilitation evolved into a more broadly focused multidisciplinary approach (e.g., Lewis, 1966; Lewin, 1968). By the 1970s, it was finally recognized that residual behavioral and cognitive impairments were the fundamental obstacles to readjustment following TBI (Richardson, 1990; Walker, 1972). This realization led to the adoption of more holistic interventions and to a shift of emphasis in rehabilitation toward the psychosocial sequelae of TBI (Forssmann-Falck & Christian, 1989; Wagner et al., 1990). Currently, there are numerous approaches to TBI rehabilitation, each approach tending to focus more or less on one or another sequela.

COGNITIVE APPROACHES

The historical roots of cognitive rehabilitation can be found in the early work of Flourens, Lashley, Goldstein, Zangwill, and Luria (Klonoff et al., 1989). During the 1940s, these researchers suggested that recovery of cerebral function may be possible. Recovery was hypothesized to be mediated through mechanisms such as substitution, direct retraining, and compensation (Zangwill, 1947). The research of this era was primarily theoretical (J. M. Stern & B. Stern, 1989); however, in 1964, Yehuda Ben-Yishay arrived at New York University and began cognitive rehabilitation applying these theories (Gordon & Hibbard, 1992; Kirn, 1987). More recently, there has been an explosion in the number of cognitive rehabilitation programs for TBI. A survey of rehabilitation units in California revealed that over 95% are currently utilizing cognitive rehabilitation techniques (Molloy, 1983).

This interest in cognitive rehabilitation is worldwide [e.g., in Italy (Zanobio, 1987) and Norway (Reinvang, 1987)]. Interestingly, it has been the concepts of Zangwill (1947) of cognitive retraining and compensation that have been most widely applied as cognitive rehabilitation techniques.

Cognitive Retraining

Cognitive retraining, also known as cognitive remediation, is based upon the hypothesis that restoration of function can occur at a neuronal level with repeated exercise on cognitive tasks (Benedict, 1989). The usual retraining protocol involves repetitive practice of tasks thought to be related to the area of cognitive impairment (e.g., memorizing lists to improve memory functioning). Computers are often used in retraining, as they present stimuli in a precise manner, are less labor-intensive, and can automatically record the trainees' scores (Molloy, 1983). The efficacy of cognitive remediation has now been called into question, however, and expression of concern about its usefulness is widespread (e.g., Berrol, 1990; Ponsford & Kinsella, 1988; Prigatano, 1987b; Zahara & Cuvo, 1984), especially when it is applied to improving memory ability (e.g., Sohlberg & Mateer, 1989; Szekeres et al., 1987). It has even been said that TBI individuals are being "encouraged to waste their time doing banal and fruitless exercises" (Robertson, Gray, & McKenzie, 1988, p. 152). In contrast, other authors claim that cognitive remediation has "come into its own as a viable form of intervention" with "numerous studies documenting its effectiveness" (Gordon & Hibbard, 1992, p. 362).

Most studies utilizing cognitive remediation have targeted either memory or attention deficits. Typical of the remediation approach to memory deficits are the papers by Ethier, Baribeau, and Braun (1989a,b). In these studies, computerized memory tasks were practiced for 4 hours each week during a period of 6 months. The 22 TBI patients who participated demonstrated statistically significant improvement on 25% of the psychometric measures utilized. In the second study, the performance of the individuals with brain injuries was significantly improved on 41% of the outcome measures. These results are characteristic of the field, the documented improvements being moderate and occurring only in a subset of the tests that have been used as outcome measures. Unfortunately, many studies in the area are flawed by lack of control groups, failure to consider improvement due to practice effects, poor generalization or maintenance of intervention gains, and the use of practice tasks as outcome measures (Niemann, Ruff, & Baser, 1990).

Research on the remediation of attention deficits appears more promising (Benedict, 1989). In 1987, Sohlberg and Mateer (1987) published a study that employed a multiple baseline design with two TBI individuals to evaluate a computer retraining program called "Attention Process Training" (APT). Both subjects improved their performance on the Paced Auditory Serial-Addition Task, a measure of attentional ability. Improvement occurred only when APT was introduced and not during memory or visual-processing retraining. Gray and Robertson (1989) obtained similar results with three TBI subjects who received computerized training designed to improve working memory. Again, improvement was specific to working memory and not to reaction time or other aspects of memory functioning. However, Gray and Robertson's results are compromised by their use of subjects who were in the very early phase after injury. At that point, the improvement in working memory could possibly reflect the normal recovery process.

The two group studies utilizing cognitive retraining for attention problems have been published. Niemann et al. (1990) randomly assigned subjects either to attention retraining or to memory retraining. The attention-retraining group improved significantly more than the memory-retraining group on all measures of attention and memory. However, there was no difference between groups on the measures of generalization. In the second study by Ben-Yishay, Piasetsky, and Rattok (1987a), 40 subjects received the "Orientation Remediation Module" (for a procedural description see Piasetsky, Ben-Yishay, Weinberg, & Diller, 1982). Subjects demonstrated significant improvement on the four measures of generalization. Five subjects were followed up 6 months later, and these subjects had maintained their improvement.

Despite such promising findings, attention retraining has not been universally found to be effective. Ponsford and Kinsella (1988) found that their TBI clients had only a 30% chance of showing improvement in attention with cognitive retraining, and then only if retraining was combined with behavioral techniques. Similarly, Wood and Fussey (1987) demonstrated that after attention retraining, subjects improved only on the practice tasks and on the behavioral measures of attention (e.g., focused eye gaze), and not on other neuropsychological measures of attention.

Cognitive retraining has also been applied to the amelioration of behavioral and emotional disturbances. This application is based upon the notion that cognitive impairment causes an inability to self-monitor and to develop and retrieve behavioral rules. These impairments then cause behavioral problems as TBI individuals violate social rules (e.g., talk too loud) and are not able to monitor and regulate their own behavior. Following from this rationale, retraining cognitive functions should ameliorate behavioral and emotional disturbances. The chapter by Malec (1984) provides a good example of this strategy. As yet, no evaluation of these methods has been published. Because the cognitive retraining is usually combined with a psychosocial intervention (e.g., social skills training), it is extremely difficult to identify which component of the intervention package has been effective.

Compensatory Approaches

In 1987, O'Connor and Cermack (1987) stated that compensatory approaches concede the irrecoverable loss of function and assist individuals to use strategies that circumvent impaired functions. Hence, the underlying assumption of compensatory approaches is that the focus should be on strengths and skills, rather than on amelioration of deficits (Kreutzer, Gordon, & Wehman, 1989). Compensation techniques are either internal, in the form of new strategies to enhance cognitive performance (e.g., the use of mnemonic techniques), or external, in the form of information-storage systems (e.g., diaries).

The teaching of new internal cognitive strategies is a common and well-researched approach. Recent studies by Cancelliere et al. (1991), Lawson and Rice (1989), Sohlberg, White, Evans, and Mateer (1992), and Wilson (1987) have involved teaching TBI individuals a wide range of techniques such as paired associate learning, the PQRST method (described in Chapter 3), prospective memory training, visual imagery, and verbal mediation techniques. Findings from these research studies and others reveal that such techniques result in improved performance on training tasks for some individuals with TBI.

However, generalization of gains to everyday memory performance seldom occurs (Godfrey & Knight, 1987), possibly because external prompts are necessary to remind individuals to use the strategies. Some increase in generalization seems to occur if self-instructional training is added as a component of intervention (e.g., Lawson & Rice, 1989). The internal strategies appear to be useful for only a restricted range of specific tasks, as they require considerable vigilance and planning to be practically useful, and they place heavy demands on cognitive systems (Benedict, 1989; O'Connor & Cermack, 1987; Sohlberg & Mateer, 1989; Zencius, Wesolowski, Krankowski, & Burke, 1991).

Use of external memory aids is the second type of compensatory approach. Memory aids include devices for storing information (e.g., notebooks), methods of cueing action (e.g., alarms, notice boards), and the use of structured environments (e.g., standardized placement of objects). While these techniques are almost universally employed, surprisingly little research has been undertaken to evaluate the efficacy of these strategies. Sohlberg and Mateer (1989) present a comprehensive three-stage approach to teach a profoundly impaired TBI person to use a diary. Diary use was established and maintained at 6 months after discharge. Using a multiple-baseline design, Burke et al. (1991) successfully aided two TBI clients with memory for work-related tasks. Finally, Zencius et al. (1991) demonstrated that providing memory notebooks with prompts led to improvement in completion of homework assignments for four TBI patients. As with cognitive strategy training, the use of memory aids does have drawbacks. Memory aids are vulnerable to damage, misplacement, or neglect (Sohlberg et al., 1992), and generalization across settings can be problematic (O'Connor & Cermack, 1987).

Combined Retraining and Compensatory Approaches

In the majority of rehabilitation settings, intervention combines retraining techniques, compensatory techniques, and education, and the intervention is administered on either an individual or a group basis (e.g., Wilson & Moffat, 1984). A wide range of cognitive functions are targeted, with a strong emphasis upon memory and attention. Surprisingly, there are few reports of interventions for executive functioning (e.g., Craine, 1982). Evaluations of intervention packages that combine cognitive retraining and compensatory approaches are very favorable. Early studies (e.g., Grafman, 1984) demonstrated moderate success, and by the 1980s, consistently positive results were being reported. For example, the TBI individuals in the study of Harrington and Levandowski (1987) improved significantly on all but one of the scales of the Luria Nebraska neuropsychological battery. In 1989, Ruff et al. (1989) assigned 40 subjects either to psychosocial intervention or to a combined cognitive retraining and compensation intervention. Both groups achieved significant improvement in their neuropsychological functioning after intervention. However, those who received the cognitive rehabilitation scored significantly higher than their controls on verbal learning and selective memory tasks. Consistent with this result, Freeman, Mittenberg, Dicowden, and Bat-Ami (1992) found significant improvement on retention of verbally presented information for a group who received both cognitive retraining and compensatory training, compared to a matched no-intervention control group.

A 5- to 10-year follow-up of participants in a memory rehabilitation program that utilized retraining and compensation found that 32% of individuals had further improvements in memory functioning, 56% had maintained the gains made during intervention, and only 12% had deteriorated (Wilson, 1992). Interestingly, the combined interventions appear to have a generalized effect. Overall improvement in cognitive functioning has been found to occur, regardless of the original function that was targeted (e.g., Middleton, Lambert, & Seggar, 1991).

Summary Comments

The adverse effects of impaired neuropsychological functioning provide a strong rationale for cognitive rehabilitation following TBI. Yet at present, the efficacy of various approaches is not convincing. Combined retraining and compensation approaches would appear to be the most promising intervention. However, as many researchers have commented, methodological problems have undermined the validity of research findings (e.g., Benedict, 1989; Gordon, 1987; Gray & Robertson, 1989). Many studies use heterogeneous patient samples, nonrandom assignment of subjects to intervention conditions, and controlled evaluation on training tasks only, and fail to control for multiple statistical comparisons (Niemann et al., 1990). As a result, it is difficult to reach any firm conclusions about the efficacy of cognitive rehabilitation approaches. In addition, the field of cognitive rehabilitation has yet to deal with its major challenge, the issue of generalization of intervention effects. Generalization from structured environments to everyday life is rare (Benedict, 1989; Diller, 1989; Kreutzer et al., 1989; Wood & Fussey, 1987). This rarity is particularly true for computer-based tasks (Berrol, 1990). Until generalization of intervention effects has been convincingly documented, the long-term benefits of cognitive rehabilitation will remain in question.

BEHAVIORAL APPROACHES

As previously outlined, TBI can result in behavioral disorders. These disorders may be very severe, involving kicking, punching, spitting, shouting, and using profane or obscene language (e.g., Turner, Green, & Braunling-McMorrow, 1990). Behavioral problems occur primarily in those TBI individuals who have experienced more severe injuries, and such problems can markedly disrupt rehabilitation, in extreme cases leaving rehabilitation staff unwilling to offer services to clients. For many years, similar behavioral problems in individuals with autism, intellectual handicap, and schizophrenia have been alleviated using behavior modification techniques (Haffey & Scibak, 1989). However, reports of the application of behavior modification to persons with TBI did not appear until the 1970s (e.g., Hollon, 1973).

Since the 1970s, behavior modification has been used with TBI individuals to eliminate unwanted problem behavior, to shape existing behavior into more appropriate forms, and to increase behavioral productivity (Gloag, 1985). The methods employed have been very similar across the studies that have evaluated this approach. The usual procedure entails careful assessment, monitoring, and functional analysis of the behavioral problem. This procedure is then followed by the use of behavior modification techniques such as differential reinforcement, time out, contingent punishment, overcorrection, and massed practice (e.g., Burke, Wesolowski, & Lane, 1988b; Wesolowski & Zencius, 1994). Some researchers have also paid attention to the maintenance of behavior change through the use of fading out of contingencies and generalization programming (e.g., Eames & Wood, 1984).

The advantages of the behavioral approach for TBI individuals are numerous. The emphasis is on real-life situations, clear goals are set, and convincing evaluation of efficacy is possible (Giles & Fussey, 1988). If successful, behavior modification can also circumvent the need for medication and its negative side effects (Haffey & Scibak, 1989). However, the application of behavior modification techniques to TBI rehabilitation has been relatively limited. While rehabilitation programs include behavioral approaches, these approaches are often seen to be merely supplementary (McGlynn, 1990), and most of the literature evaluating the use of behavior modification techniques with TBI individuals is in the form of single-case AB designs. The lack of utilization of behavioral technology may be due to the misconception that behavioral techniques will be ineffective with the TBI population, who are characterized by difficulty in learning and slowness in information processing (G. Goldstein & Ruthven, 1983). However, even seriously debilitated individuals are able to learn new associations (McGlynn, 1990), and behavior modification is extremely successful with those with severe intellectual retardation (G. Goldstein & Ruthven, 1983; Tate, 1987a).

It has also been argued that behavioral disorders are organically caused and therefore will not respond to interventions that simply control the environment (e.g., Tate, 1987b). Nonetheless, it is apparent that not all behavior disorders can be attributable to organic damage (Wood, 1987). It is also true that etiology does not necessarily determine the nature of successful intervention. The literature in the area of the application of behavior modification to problems following TBI is briefly reviewed below.

Modification of Behavioral Excesses

Researchers have published a considerable number of single-case intervention studies that document the effectiveness of applications of behavior modification procedures with TBI individuals. The most common behavioral excesses targeted in these studies are aggressive behavior (Godfrey & Knight, 1988; Hollon, 1973; Horton & Howe, 1981; L. C. Peters et al., 1992; Tate, 1987a; Turner et al., 1990; Wood, 1987) and verbal outbursts (Alderman, 1991; Burke & Lewis, 1986; Hegel, 1988; Wood, 1987); however, behavior modification has also been applied with disruptive behavior (Burke & Wesolowski, 1988), self-injurious behavior (M. D. Peters, Gluck, & McCormick, 1992), and sexualized behavior (Wood, 1988b). In general, results have been favorable, although it has been found that aggressive outbursts do not respond well to extinction techniques (Burke et al., 1988b).

The main limitation of research on the application of behavior modification techniques to the amelioration of behavioral excesses is that most of the successful interventions have been carried out in highly structured inpatient settings. Application of behavior modification procedures in the home environment may be problematic, as families may not have the skills or emotional resources to manage behavioral problems with detachment (DeFazio, Kelly, & Flynn, 1989). The psychological status of family members can also result in inconsistent responses to TBI behavior (Tate, 1987b), thereby undermining behavioral intervention, which relies on consistency of appropriate responses to target behaviors. Wood (1988b) has attempted to apply behavioral techniques in a day hospital. He notes that the daily change of environment from home to hospital presents a major obstacle to improvement in behavioral functioning and that interventions rely on the understanding and cooperation of family members. Generalization does not necessarily occur, even within settings in the hospital environment (e.g., Hegel, 1988). Consequently, specific programming (e.g., the training of exemplars) is being developed to overcome this problem (Haffey & Scibak, 1989; McGlynn, 1990; Zahara & Cuvo, 1984).

Modification of Behavioral Deficits

Modifying behavioral deficits tends to be more problematic, and less effective, than modifying behavioral excesses (Wood, 1984). Self-care skills such as dressing and grooming can be taught, but increasing the overall behavioral productivity of a TBI individual may be more difficult. Motivational problems often fail to respond to the use of rewards, as it can be very difficult to identify effective reinforcers for the TBI individual (Haffey & Scibak, 1989). According to Wood and Burgess (1988), the difficulty in identifying effective reinforcers is that frontal damage reduces the victim's sense of pleasure; consequently, the amount of effort that is required to initiate an action is perceived as being excessive for the intrinsic value of the reinforcer. These authors recommend creating appropriate habits through the process of overlearning, so that performance of behaviors becomes associated with external cues. Spontaneous appropriate behavior is also rewarded, and shaping is used to teach complex behaviors as part of behavior modification programs (Eames & Wood, 1984). To date, research has not demonstrated that behavior modification procedures result in improved motivation as reflected in more generalized increases in goal-directed behavior.

Modification of Cognitive Deficits

Behavioral techniques have also been utilized to improve cognitive functions such as memory and attention (e.g., G. Goldstein & Ruthven, 1983). Fowler, Hart, and Sheehan (1972) report a study in which a male with TBI improved his ability to keep appointments on time when he was reinforced for doing so or ignored when he was late. At 15 months follow-up, this effect was maintained. Attention-related behaviors such as time on task and eye contact have also been found to be trainable (Benedict, 1989; Gray & Robertson, 1989; Wood, 1984, 1987). More recently, a controlled study by Deacon and Campbell (1991) indicated that the use of feedback and cues improves choice reaction time to near-normal performance levels. However, it is doubtful whether behavior modification has any direct impact on cognitive abilities such as short-term verbal memory or speed of information processing. The best approach to improving cognitive functioning would appear to be a combination of both cognitive and behavioral techniques.

Summary Comments

Behavioral technology has been utilized in TBI rehabilitation for many years. However, the application of behavior modification techniques has tended to be restricted to a few rehabilitation programs that specialize in the management of serious behavioral disorders. Empirically, the approach appears to have great potential, but there is a need for well-designed research that pays careful attention to factors such as accurate sample description, the use of objective measures of behavior change, the use of multiple-baseline designs, and assessment of generalization and maintenance (McGlynn, 1990). More attention must also be paid to the amelioration of behavioral deficits. Motivational problems as reflected in a generalized lowering of goal-directed behavior are among the most difficult obstacles to readjustment following TBI. Unfortunately, our knowledge of how to effectively manage motivational problems is sorely inadequate.

PSYCHOTHERAPEUTIC APPROACHES

Following TBI, individuals are faced with the monumental task of matching their preinjury self-image to the new reality (Florian et al., 1991; Gordon & Hibbard, 1992). Enormous adjustments in expectations and life-styles are required. Yet the deficits in cognition and behavior make readjustment problematic (Florian et al., 1991). TBI sufferers' struggle to adapt often results in the development of inappropriate coping strategies (Letoff, 1983). When inappropriate coping strategies are combined with neuropsychologically mediated personality disturbances and emotional reactions to loss, a complex psychological picture evolves. Psychotherapy may be vital if reasonable readjustment is to be accomplished (Cicerone, 1989; Prigatano, 1987a).

However, individuals with TBI have traditionally been considered poor candidates for psychotherapy because of the effect cognitive and neurobehavioral sequelae have upon insight and the ability to learn (Gobble, Henry, Pfahl, & Smith, 1987; Gordon & Hibbard, 1992; Rosenthal, 1989). Rehabilitation programs emphasize cognitive retraining, while emotional problems tend to be haphazardly dealt with (Prigatano et al., 1984). Nevertheless, psychotherapeutic approaches are gaining wider acceptance, particularly since the late 1980s. Intervention approaches are being tailored with greater sophistication. Therapists are required to be well versed in TBI (Rosenthal, 1989), and directive counseling approaches are increasingly being emphasized (Gobble et al., 1987).

It has also become apparent that successful interventions are not related as much to theoretical models of therapy as to factors such as empathy, repetitive feedback, and ability to motivate clients (Cicerone, 1989; Prigatano et al., 1986; Rosenthal, 1989). The use of group therapy is also increasing because of its usefulness in providing social-behavior feedback and its ability to provide a context for practicing interpersonal skills (Gobble et al., 1987). Forssmann-Falck and Christian (1989) provide a good review of the use of group psychotherapy following TBI, and Prigatano et al. (1986a) describe an exemplary psychotherapy group in their paper. The literature in the area of psychotherapy following TBI is reviewed below. Unfortunately, very little empirical research has been carried out on psychotherapy for TBI, and most studies are purely descriptive. The need for research in this area is obvious and has been noted by many authors (e.g., Rosenthal, 1989).

Dynamic Psychotherapy

The literature in this field is extremely scant, although there are some published descriptive reports of dynamic psychotherapy with TBI individuals. The majority of this work has been carried out in Israel by Stern and colleagues (Geva & Stern, 1985; J. M. Stern, 1985; B. Stern & J. M. Stern, 1985; Tadir & Stern, 1985). Their approach involves the use of dream therapy as a means of circumventing denial, grief therapy to address loss issues, and Freudian therapy for the reconciliation of aggressive and libidinal drives. The efficacy of their techniques has been evaluated by using anecdotal case reports. The results of these anecdotal case reports are invariably favorable. Morris and Bleiberg (1986) report the use of dynamic psychotherapy with a 31-year-old male with TBI whose intellectual functioning remained intact. Therapy reportedly had a positive outcome, the man involved improving his work functioning and being promoted to a more senior work position. However, a multicomponent intervention was employed, with relaxation and cognitive training also being utilized. Other authors have also employed similar intervention packages with reported success (e.g., D. W. Ellis, 1989; Glassman, 1991).

Unfortunately, the use of multiple techniques as part of a program makes it difficult to partial out the efficacy of dynamic psychotherapy alone. Dynamic psychotherapy for TBI individuals has tended to involve attempts to reconcile preinjury and present self-image. For instance, Muir and Haffey (1984) refer to the reconciliation of preinjury and present selves as "mobile mourning," while Morris and Bleiberg (1986) discuss recovery from "narcissistic injury." The infrequency of reports of the use of dynamic psychotherapy is most probably due to the difficulty TBI individuals have with the higher mental functions upon which dynamic psychotherapy relies.

Cognitive–Behavioral Therapy

According to Cicerone (1989), cognitive–behavioral techniques are readily applicable to subjects with TBI, as these techniques tend to be relatively structured and directive. Predictably, very little research has been carried out in this area. This research is reviewed below under the specific techniques that were utilized.

Relaxation Training

Relaxation training has been employed to assist TBI individuals in coping with situationally related stress (e.g., anxiety in the workplace). Lysaght and Bodenhamer (1990) taught four clients biofeedback, autogenic relaxation, and deep breathing. Outcome was assessed using electromyographic profiles and scores on the Sickness Impact Profile. Clients in this study did achieve lowered levels of physiological arousal during sessions, but scores at 4-week follow-up were not significantly different from preintervention scores.

Problem-Solving Training

There are many anecdotal reports on problem-solving training in the literature, with few controlled evaluations of its efficacy. Foxx, Marchand-Martella, Martella, Braunling-McMorrow, and McMorrow (1988) and Foxx, Martella, and Marchand-Martella (1989) describe a method of teaching problem solving by the use of cue cards, response-specific feedback, modeling, self-monitoring, positive reinforcement, response practice, and self-correction. Three TBI adults undertook this training in applied problem solving in areas such as transportation, safety, and medication. Compared to a matched no-intervention control group of TBI individuals, the intervention group were better able to solve problems in the targeted areas. Although this approach is promising, the paucity of outcome data makes it difficult to draw any firm conclusions about the efficacy of problem-solving training from these studies.

Stress-Inoculation Training

Stress-inoculation procedures are beginning to become a popular choice of intervention for the management of aggression following TBI. Lira, Carne, and Masri (1983) provide an example of a typical stress-inoculation program that involved cognitive preparation, skills acquisition, and application training. In their case study, a 22-year-old male reduced his number of aggressive outbursts from 2.75 per week to 0.5 per week. At 5-month follow-up, frequency of outbursts had further reduced to zero. Extended stress-inoculation programs that include problem solving, redirection, and inconvenience reviews have also proved successful (e.g., Burke et al., 1988b; McKinlay & Hickox, 1988).

Rational Emotive Therapy

Rational emotive therapy is not commonly used with TBI patients because of the cognitive demands of its cognitive restructuring technique. However, Malec (1984) presents an anecdotal case study of the successful use of rational emotive therapy with a female who became depressed after sustaining a TBI. Pleasant-events scheduling was implemented along with the cognitive modification designed to ameliorate negative thought patterns.

Self-Instructional Training

Self-instructional training has been found to be successful in ameliorating affective and behavioral problems following TBI (Cicerone, 1989). However, the majority of the reports of the use of self-instructional training involve training in cognitive task performance. Barry and Riley (1987) utilized self-instructional training to improve performance on the Kaufman Hand Movements Test, and Cicerone and Wood (1987) applied it to the Tower of London Task. Robertson et al. (1988) used self-instructional training to improve performance on visual neglect tasks, and Webster and Scott (1983) employed this technique to improve performance on the story memory test. The application of self-instructional training strategies to cognitive functioning has been moderately successful, with gains being maintained at follow-up. The use of self-instructional training within this context is based upon Luria's hypothesis that attention in normal adults is mediated by inner speech (Webster & Scott, 1983). Self-instructional training has also been employed to improve interpersonal problem solving (Cicerone & Wood, 1987); however, no systematic evaluation of its efficacy in this area has been carried out. A major drawback of self-instructional training is that it requires self-monitoring abilities that may be impaired following TBI (McGlynn, 1990).

Psychosexual Intervention

Descriptions of psychosexual interventions following TBI are virtually nonexistent. Burke et al. (1991) report having successfully reduced exhibitionism using a self-control program, and Blackerby (1990) describes a model multifaceted program with social-skills role plays, education, sensate focus exercises, and reassurance. According to Blackerby (1990), his program is not fully implemented at any rehabilitation facility and has not been empirically evaluated.

Interpersonal-Skills Training

Interpersonal-skills training is the most commonly implemented cognitive behavioral intervention subsequent to TBI. The reason is probably that deficits in interpersonal functioning have a widespread impact on social role functioning

(Helffenstein & Wechsler, 1982). Many of the early interpersonal-skills training interventions were purely behavioral in focus; however, attention is now being paid to the way in which people perceive themselves and the social situations they are in (Brotherton et al., 1988). The research on interpersonal-skills training encompasses both multiple-baseline studies (e.g., Brotherton et al., 1988; Giles et al., 1988) and group outcome studies (e.g., Helffenstein & Wechsler, 1982; D. A. Johnson & Newton, 1987). Interventions have been applied either on an individual basis (e.g., Giles & Clark-Wilson, 1988a) or in the group context (e.g., Ben-Yishay & Lakin, 1989). Frequently, techniques entail the use of simulated conversations, reciprocal games, feedback, modeling, self-monitoring, and reinforcement. Results have been mixed. Direct observation measures show little change in complex social behaviors such as reciprocation in conversations (e.g., Helffenstein & Wechsler, 1982), although some changes in simple motoric behaviors, frequency of verbalization, and number of compliments given have been noted (e.g., Braunling-McMorrow, Lloyd, & Fralish, 1986; Brotherton et al., 1988; Giles et al., 1988; Schloss, Thompson, Gajar, & Schloss, 1985). Self-report measures of anxiety and self-concept do improve with training, as do the reports of TBI clients' social skills made by relatives (e.g., Helffenstein & Wechsler, 1982). Positive findings are not universal, however, with some authors reporting no significant benefits of interpersonal-skills training (e.g., D. A. Johnson & Newton, 1987). Nevertheless, impressive gains in interactional skills have been reported in some studies (e.g., Gajar, Schloss, Schloss, & Thompson, 1984), and interventions are becoming increasingly innovative (for a description of mediational techniques, see Gross, Ben-Nahum, & Munk, 1982). Interpersonal-skills training has shown some promise; however, this intervention approach requires further development and evaluation.

Feedback Techniques

Feedback techniques are often employed to increase TBI individuals' awareness of their deficits following injury. This technique is very controversial. Some clinicians view lack of awareness as the predominant cause of low motivation during rehabilitation, failure to utilize compensatory strategies, and maintenance of unrealistic goals (Youngjohn & Altman, 1989). Because of this drawback, it is deemed necessary to promote awareness so that better outcome may be achieved (Deaton, 1986). In contrast to this view, other authors claim that increasing awareness may not be a valuable characteristic in and of itself (Cicerone, 1989; Novack & Richards, 1991) and that lack of awareness may well promote hope and well-being (Moore, Stambrook, & Peters, 1989; Ridley, 1989). The etiology of lack of awareness is also under debate, there being differing opinions regarding the extent to which lack of awareness reflects brain damage or is a psychological defense mechanism (Ben-Yishay et al., 1985).

Despite this controversy, feedback techniques are commonly used as a means of increasing awareness. Feedback is usually given either through the use of a computer, videotape, or group therapy or through performance on supervised activities (Deaton, 1986; Ylvisaker & Szekeres, 1989). The aim of feedback is to provide the patient with a means whereby self-perception can be tested against others' perceptions of reality. There has been very little research on the effectiveness of feedback techniques because of the difficulty of operationally defining what awareness actually is. The measurement of awareness has usually involved comparison of the TBI individuals' evaluation of their functioning with that of relatives or health professionals or with their actual performance (e.g., Allen & Ruff, 1990).

Thus, Fordyce and Roueche (1986) describe a study in which TBI individuals were allocated into groups on the basis of their level of awareness of deficits as measured by comparison with staff perceptions. After education, video feedback, group-based feedback, and reinforcement of behaviors indicative of self-acceptance, some TBI individuals' ratings became more consistent with those of staff. Youngjohn and Altman (1989) found similar results when persons with brain injuries were asked to predict performance on cognitive tasks and then given feedback publicly after the task was completed. Interestingly, some of the clients in this study displayed mild reactive depression in response to the feedback. Feedback would appear to be most effective when it is given in the context of a working therapeutic alliance and balances confrontation and support (Ben-Yishay et al., 1985; Cicerone, 1989; Klonoff et al., 1989).

Family-Based Interventions

The role of family members in rehabilitation is paramount. Involving the family fosters positive dynamics within the family system, provides information that helps to further delineate the TBI individual's problems, increases the chances of generalization of skills, and enhances the TBI individual's progress (Mauss-Clum & Ryan, 1981; McKinlay & Hickox, 1988; Rogers & Kreutzer, 1984; Rosenthal, 1989). At present, the primary approach to family intervention is that of providing education. Studies in the 1970s and 1980s indicated that families were unhappy with the amount of education offered (e.g., Mauss-Clum & Ryan, 1981; Oddy et al., 1978a; Panting & Merry, 1972), and very little written information was available at that time (Eisner & Kreutzer, 1989). However, a multitude of education programs have now been developed (e.g., Rao, Sulton, Young, & Harvey, 1986) in the belief that families who understand the effects of TBI will be better able to cope (Grinspun, 1987; J. R. Johnson & Higgins, 1987; Klonoff & Prigatano, 1987). Evaluation of education programs is complex, as so many factors affect long-term outcome that it can be difficult to single out the specific effects of an educational program that is but one part of a multicomponent rehabilitation program (Grinspun, 1987). Sanguinetti and Catanzaro (1987) describe a study in which 9 families received education on neurophysical sequelae while 29 families received information on cognitive dysfunction. The latter group performed better on a test that required them to answer how they would respond to real TBI-related problems in six different scenarios. These findings provide some support for the utility of educational approaches.

Other family-based interventions include family therapy, family support groups, and family counseling, but to date, outcome research has failed to demonstrate that the TBI individual's long-term prognosis is improved by these interventions (Rosenthal, 1984). Hegeman (1988) provides a typical example of family-based intervention, and many other descriptions of such programs have been published (e.g., Anderson & Parente, 1985; Durgin, 1989; Shaw & McMahon, 1990; Soderstrom et al., 1988). Lezak (1986) presents an interesting six-stage model of family therapy that has great heuristic value in guiding clinical practice. It is encouraging to note that interventions for families of TBI individuals are now beginning to include the teaching of problem-solving skills (e.g., Jacobs, 1989) and emphasize networking within the community (e.g., Rogers & Kreutzer, 1984). Only two studies have been published examining the utility of involving the family in assisting with the TBI individual's rehabilitation program. One of these studies failed to include a no-intervention control comparison (McKinlay & Hickox, 1988), and the other suggested that high levels of involvement on the part of the family may prove overly burdensome (Quine, Pierce, & Lyle, 1988).

Summary Comments

There is little doubt that TBI individuals face a wide range of difficulties in the months and years following their injuries. These difficulties can prove very distressing and require TBI individuals and their families to make major adjustments in their life-styles and expectations. The need for psychotherapy in such circumstances is often apparent. Fortunately, knowledge concerning the use of psychotherapeutic techniques after TBI is increasing, and cognitive behavioral therapy, family-based interventions, and group psychotherapy all seem promising. However, the lack of intervention-outcome research prevents the drawing of definitive conclusions regarding the efficacy of any form of psychotherapy for TBI individuals. There is an urgent need for controlled outcome studies that evaluate the effectiveness of the various psychotherapeutic interventions available.

PSYCHOPHARMACOLOGICAL APPROACHES

Prompted by findings of altered neurotransmitter balances following TBI, a range of psychopharmacological treatments have been utilized (Lal, Merbitz, &

Grip, 1988; Weinberg, Auerbach, & Moore, 1987). Use of anticonvulsants in the treatment of posttraumatic epilepsy is now standard practice (R. W. Evans, Gualtieri, & Patterson, 1987), and psychotropic medication is increasingly being administered to ameliorate behavioral problems, affective disorders, and cognitive deficits following TBI. Various pharmacological agents such as midazolam (Wroblewski & Joseph, 1992), amitriptyline (Jackson, Corrigan, & Arnett, 1985; Mysiw & Jackson, 1987), propranolol (Yudofsky, Williams, & Gorman, 1981), and carbamazepine (McAllister, 1985) have been recommended for the treatment of aggressive behavior and irritability in TBI individuals. Similarly, tricyclic antidepressants have been recommended for the treatment of depression following TBI (e.g., Jackson et al., 1985; Mysiw & Jackson, 1987), even though tricyclics have been found to be relatively unsuccessful in alleviating depression following minor head injury (Dinan & Mobayed, 1992).

With respect to the amelioration of cognitive deficits, experimental work is being carried out using psychostimulants (e.g., vasopressin, physostigmine) in a manner similar to their use with hyperactive children. Some single-case studies indicate that this approach may have potential (e.g., R. W. Evans et al., 1987; Weinberg et al., 1987); however, the findings by Gualtieri and Evans (1988), who employed a double-blind placebo control design, were not favorable. The lack of treatment-outcome research for drug treatments makes it difficult to reach a conclusion about the effectiveness of psychostimulants at this time (Richardson, 1990).

As with so many other approaches to rehabilitation following TBI, the lack of controlled outcome research in the area of pharmacological treatment is startling (Cope, 1987). Studies have been published that failed to include a control condition, lacked objective outcome measures, and ignored spontaneous recovery (e.g., Jackson et al., 1985; Lipper & Tuchman, 1976). Differences among studies in their sample characteristics, dosage of medication, and route of administration are also common, making comparisons across studies difficult. Authors also extrapolate freely from research involving other types of brain injuries such as cardiovascular accidents (e.g., Mysiw, Jackson, & Corrigan, 1988) and from animal studies (e.g., O'Shanick, 1988). Given the nature and complexity of neurological damage following TBI, this extrapolation may not be justified.

The issue of drug side effects is also of concern. The literature contains reports that pharmacological agents such as fluoxetine and desipramine lowered the threshold for seizures and resulted in increased seizure activity in TBI individuals (e.g., Wroblewski, Guidos, Leary, & Joseph, 1992). Control of such behavior may also be established at the expense of reduced adaptive functioning (Cope, 1987). This outcome is particularly likely with neuroleptic medications (Jackson et al., 1985). Paradoxical increases in agitation and unacceptable sedation have occurred with the use of neuroleptics (Mysiw & Jackson, 1987), and a recent study demonstrated significant functional improvements in a TBI patient whose medication was tapered off and replaced with behavioral interventions (Cantini, Gluck, & McLean, 1992).

Summary Comments

A large range of psychopharmacological treatments for TBI-related problems have been employed. However, the results of treatment-outcome studies in this area are equivocal with respect to the ability of these pharmaceutical agents to improve the mood, behavior, and cognitive functioning of TBI individuals. Moreover, these drugs have a number of potentially harmful side effects. Because of the equivocal advantage of medication use, and the potential side effects, psychopharmacological treatment for TBI sequelae other than epilepsy and agitation during acute treatment should be employed with caution.

VOCATIONAL REHABILITATION

The majority of TBI victims are males under the age of 25 (Kreutzer et al., 1991). Men in this age group would normally expect to have many years of productive work life ahead of them. It is not surprising, therefore, that considerable effort has been devoted to the vocational rehabilitation of patients with TBI. There are several different models of the delivery of vocational rehabilitation services. Vocational rehabilitation services can operate as programs in their own right (e.g., Gobble et al., 1987), as one component of multicomponent programs (e.g., Ben-Yishay et al., 1985), or on an individualized outpatient basis (e.g., DePoy, 1987). Programs typically include assessment, vocational therapy (i.e., behavior modification, cognitive rehabilitation, interpersonal-skills training), counseling, work conditioning, job training, and job placement (e.g., Haffey & Lewis, 1989; Smith, 1983).

Uncontrolled studies of vocational rehabilitation programs indicate positive outcomes. For example, Wehman and colleagues have used the "supported employment" approach, which provides vocational intervention at the point of job placement through the use of a job coach. Their research shows positive gains associated with vocational rehabilitation, including an increase in amount of money earned and the number of hours worked (Kreutzer et al., 1988, 1989, 1991; Wehman et al., 1989a–c). Cost–benefit analysis of supported employment has also been favorable (West et al., 1991). However, supported employment has not always been found to be successful. There are failures to return to work following TBI, although usually only on the part of very severely disabled victims. Other uncontrolled studies of vocational rehabilitation programs also report positive results (e.g., Ben-Yishay et al., 1985, 1987b; Jellinek & Harvey, 1982; Lyons & Morse, 1988; Simon, 1988). Unfortunately, interpretation of this research is hampered by the varying definitions of "return to work," which have included full-time paid positions, looking after children at home, doing volunteer work, or being placed in a sheltered workshop.

To date, two controlled outcome studies evaluating vocational rehabilitation have been published. In the first, the employment rates of TBI individuals in a work-reentry program were compared to those of TBI individuals who received either inpatient or day hospital rehabilitation that did not target return to work (Haffey & Abrams, 1991). Of the work-reentry participants, 68% were placed in jobs, compared to 34% and 39% of the inpatient and day rehabilitation groups, respectively. However, 50% of the work-reentry placements were not sustained, and no statistical comparisons between groups were reported for the follow-up assessments. In the second study, TBI individuals either received a multicomponent intervention program or were part of a no-intervention control group (Prigatano et al., 1984). The multicomponent intervention aimed to improve vocational skills, but did not include actual work trials. Of the intervention group, 50% were working at follow-up (ranging from 8 to 33 months after discharge) as compared to 36% of the no-intervention group. This outcome was not as successful as expected; consequently, occupational trials were introduced into the intervention program. When this revised program was evaluated, 45% of those TBI individuals who had occupational placements were working at follow-up compared to 49% of those who did not receive the trials (see Haffey & Lewis, 1989). Such findings cast doubt on the efficacy of occupational trials.

Summary Comments

Vocational readjustment is frequently of great personal significance to the person with TBI. This significance, coupled with the financial cost of failure to return to work [as much as $500,000 to $1 million dollars per person (Godfrey et al., 1993a)], highlights the need for effective vocational rehabilitation. Uncontrolled studies indicate positive results using program models such as supported employment. However, there are very few published controlled outcome studies. Further research is essential if the efficacy of vocational rehabilitation is to be convincingly established.

MULTICOMPONENT REHABILITATION PROGRAMS

The 1980s and 1990s have witnessed the growth of multicomponent rehabilitation programs (Levin, 1990a). In the United States alone, the number of multicomponent traumatic brain injury rehabilitation centers has expanded from

16 in 1980 to over 450 in the late 1980s (Kirn, 1987). The increased availability of advocacy organizations, the general trend for psychologists to be more involved in health care, and the steady rise in TBI incidence and survival rates have all contributed to this expansion (Trexler, 1987).

The multicomponent rehabilitation programs that have been developed typically incorporate a wide range of intervention techniques that are delivered in a multidisciplinary context. The combination of cognitive approaches with psychotherapy and vocational training is common. Ironically, many programs are labeled as "cognitive rehabilitation" despite their obvious multicomponent approach (e.g., Fryer & Haffey, 1987; Mills, Nesbeda, Katz, & Alexander, 1992). Although the initial emphasis of multicomponent rehabilitation programs was on comprehensive medically based residential programs, the current trend is for day hospital programs. Those TBI patients with very severe deficits are now referred to community reentry programs or transitional living centers (Uomoto & McLean, 1989). The reentry programs or transitional living centers are community-based residential homes staffed by multidisciplinary health care workers. Unfortunately, studies examining the efficacy of multicomponent programs are rare (Editorial, 1990; Giles & Fussey, 1988). Indeed, this lack of intervention-outcome research has been described by one author as "outrageous" (Richardson, 1990). The outcome literature on postacute multicomponent rehabilitation is reviewed below.

Inpatient Multicomponent Rehabilitation Programs

Only three controlled evaluations of inpatient programs have been published. The interpretation of the study by Gobiet (1989) is problematic due to methodological problems (e.g., unclear description of sample characteristics and assignment to conditions). The other two studies indicate that early rehabilitation can result in decreased length of admission to postacute rehabilitation hospitals without compromising long-term outcome (Cope & Hall, 1982; MacKay, Bernstein, Chapman, Morgan, & Milazzo, 1992). However, it is not clear from these studies whether early intervention resulted in improved functional outcome or whether the benefits of intervention continue once participation in the program ceases.

Uncontrolled outcome studies have documented significant improvement associated with program participation. Following participation in inpatient rehabilitation programs, TBI individuals' level of independence in living situations has been found to improve, as have scores on rating scales measuring functional abilities, psychosocial status, behavior, involvement in household management, self-care skills, client and relative stress levels, mobility, communication, and disability levels (Askensay & Rahmani, 1988; Burke et al., 1991; Eames & Wood, 1985; Fryer & Haffey, 1987; Johnston, 1991; Johnston & Lewis, 1991; Najenson et al., 1980; Panting & Merry, 1972; Ranseen, 1985; Sahgal & Heinemann, 1989).

Unfortunately, the uncontrolled nature of these studies limits the conclusions that can be drawn regarding the efficacy of multicomponent inpatient programs.

Outpatient Multicomponent Day Programs

The outpatient day hospital movement began with demonstration programs developed by Ben-Yishay et al. (1985) and Prigatano et al. (1984). The models developed in these programs have been applied in rehabilitation settings around the Western world (e.g., Christensen et al., 1992). The emphasis of these programs is holistic, and they provide intensive client contact over long time periods (e.g., 4 days a week for 6 months). Uncontrolled evaluations of multicomponent outpatient programs have generally documented significant improvements in functioning for program participants (Braun, Baribeau, & Ethier, 1988; Christensen et al., 1992; Cole, Cope, & Cervelli, 1985; Cope, Cole, Hall, & Barkan, 1991a,b; Epperson-Sebour & Rifkin, 1985; Heilbronner, Roueche, Everson, & Epler, 1989; Mills et al., 1992; Namerow, 1987; Scherzer, 1986; J. M. Stern et al., 1985). Although limited in number, controlled evaluations of multicomponent outpatient programs are very promising, having documented significant improvements on selected neuropsychological measures, on ratings of functional ability, and on personality measures, relative to no-intervention control conditions. Furthermore, this relative advantage has been maintained at follow-up assessment (G. Goldstein & Ruthven, 1983; Prigatano et al., 1984).

One of the most comprehensive controlled research studies to date is the evaluation of the Rusk Institute program (Rattok et al., 1992). In this study, TBI individuals were assigned to one of three groups that received either standard multicomponent interventions, interventions without intense cognitive rehabilitation, or interventions without small-group interactions. Results indicated no differences between the groups on the neuropsychological outcome measures. Improvements on 47% of neuropsychological tests were noted for all three groups. Groups receiving cognitive remediation did perform significantly better on some near transfer tasks (e.g., visual processing); however, all groups improved significantly over time on these tasks. No significant differences between groups were found on behavioral, interpersonal, intrapersonal, or employability measures.

Summary Comments

Although some impressive improvements in functioning have been documented in uncontrolled evaluations of multicomponent rehabilitation programs, methodological limitations associated with uncontrolled trials prevent the drawing of conclusions regarding efficacy from these studies. The studies reported are often characterized by methodological problems such as vague sample description, use of unmatched groups, variations in duration of follow-up, a restricted range of outcome measures, lack of no-intervention or waiting-list control comparison conditions, idiosyncratic definitions of outcome (e.g., the definition of return to work), and the absence of baseline and follow-up assessments. Furthermore, the extent to which improvements in neuropsychological tests and rating scales reflect clinically significant improvement remains in question.

In 1972, Walker (1972) prophetically stated (p. 156) that "the current dress of rehabilitation is only a fad." Since that time, approaches to rehabilitation following TBI have changed rapidly. The use of cognitive rehabilitation has become commonplace, and increasing focus is being placed upon behavioral and psychotherapeutic techniques. Unfortunately, research has not kept pace with application. The results of well-controlled empirical evaluations of programs are not available to allow one to assess the merits of these new rehabilitation approaches that are currently in use. Hence, with the possible exception of multicomponent day programs, for which there is encouraging preliminary evidence of efficacy, it is very difficult to reach conclusions about even the most basic of questions, such as whether rehabilitation following TBI is actually beneficial. Nevertheless, research strategies are becoming more sophisticated, and the next decade should see considerable clarification regarding the efficacy of rehabilitation methods.

3

Compensating for Cognitive Impairment

Cognitive impairment represents a major barrier to vocational, emotional, and interpersonal functioning for many individuals affected by traumatic brain injury (TBI). For example, it may be difficult to obtain a job if one is unable to formulate a plan for locating vacant positions. Similarly, it may be an onerous task to maintain friendships when one cannot remember the content of conversations. In fact, the successful completion of many activities of daily living require the very cognitive skills that are impaired following TBI. Family members are affected by a TBI victim's cognitive impairment as they grapple on a daily basis with the victim's poor judgment, forgetfulness, and limited concentration span, which are frequent problems following TBI. The TBI victim may now require constant assistance from family members in the form of prompting to remember appointments, to locate lost objects, and to make decisions.

In recognition of the impact that cognitive impairment has upon both TBI individuals and their families, the family support program provided a range of interventions designed to teach cognitive compensatory techniques. In this chapter, the theoretical basis for the compensatory model of cognitive rehabilitation is discussed, and the compensatory techniques that were employed in the family support program are described.

FUNCTIONAL ADAPTATION: A COMPENSATORY APPROACH TO COGNITIVE REHABILITATION

The compensatory approach to cognitive rehabilitation used in the family support program is based upon the functional adaptation model. Functional adaptation concedes the irrecoverable loss of cognitive function following brain injury and espouses helping victims to use alternative means to attain success at tasks that they can no longer perform in the usual manner (Wilson, 1989). Craine (1982) makes the analogy that functional adaptation is comparable to an orchestra that, when its violin players die, asks other instrumentalists to learn the violin parts. Arising from this model is an approach in which intervention aims to enhance existing skills and to adapt them to compensate for impairment. The cognitive skills that need to be improved or adapted are directly targeted by techniques such as diary use or self-instructional training. The underlying philosophy of the compensatory approach is in contrast to cognitive remediation, in which intervention aims to ameliorate deficits through the retraining of lost functions (Prigatano, 1987b). The debate concerning the relative merits of cognitive remediation vs. cognitive compensation approaches to rehabilitation is ongoing, and there is insufficient empirical evidence to reach a valid conclusion regarding the relative efficacy of either approach (see Chapter 2 for a discussion of this research).

The compensatory techniques employed in the family support program were implemented on an individual basis. Group-training interventions were precluded due to the geographic dispersal of the families in the program. However, clinical experience has indicated that cognitive compensation techniques can be effectively taught in the group context. The format of group interventions varies widely, but usually involves weekly or daily group meetings that teach skills such as mnemonic strategies, the use of memory aids, and participation in group exercises such as memory games (e.g., Wilson & Moffat, 1984). These groups are often run as part of a multicomponent rehabilitation program.

OVERCOMING MEMORY IMPAIRMENT

The presence of memory impairment in TBI individuals was reported by almost all the families in the support program. This finding is in accordance with other research results in which the majority of families have reported memory impairment in the TBI individual, even as long as 7 years after injury (Oddy et al., 1985). Approximately two thirds of the TBI individuals in the family support program identified themselves as having sustained memory impairment. Examples of memory problems demonstrated by the TBI individuals included losing keys, forgetting conversations, and being unable to recall activities undertaken during quite recent periods of time (e.g., on the two previous days). Memory problems were most readily apparent for verbal information, in particular with short-term memory for spoken communication. Neuropsychological testing of TBI patients on the Wechsler Memory Scale—Revised confirmed the clinical observation of relatively intact visual memory and impaired verbal memory for the majority of participants. The most marked impact of verbal memory impairment was upon work performance. Individuals reported being berated by employers for not correctly carrying out instructions they could not remember and feeling intensely frustrated when they were unable to remember workmates' conversations.

Families also reported that coping with the consequences of cognitive impairment could be difficult. In some cases, memory impairment caused safety problems. Susan, for example, would forget to fasten her son's seat belt. This omission eventually resulted in the child being bruised when Susan drove the car over a rough roadway. For other families, the TBI individual's lack of planning ability led to time-consuming rescue attempts to rectify the consequences of poor financial decisions and uncompleted projects. The impact of cognitive impairment was greatest for the family when the TBI individual also displayed limited awareness of cognitive impairment. Many families were faced with guiding decision making or providing prompts to a TBI individual who resented their assistance and interpreted it as implying that he was not capable of independent living. The result was often frustration on the part of all parties.

External Memory Aids

Diary Use

Because of the difficulty TBI victims have with prospective memory (i.e., memory for future events), participants in the program commonly used diaries. Diaries have the advantages that they both reduce the demand on memory by providing a permanent written record of information and provide a physical prompt for remembering information. Interestingly, in a recent follow-up study of TBI individuals who were 5–10 years postinjury, notebooks, diaries, and wall planners were in the top 10 most commonly used memory aids. Moreover, the TBI individuals were using memory strategies more frequently at follow-up than when these techniques were first taught (Wilson, 1992). Very little research has been carried out to evaluate the efficacy of diary use, but those studies that have been conducted indicate that diary use can result in rapid improvement in prospective memory performance (e.g., Zencius et al., 1991).

The procedure employed to train diary use was based on the Sohlberg and Mateer (1989) acquisition, application, and adaptation format. The use of the dictaphone and of computerized daily planners was taught by the same method as diary use. The first step was to identify the type of diary best suited to the TBI individual's requirements. Standard office diaries were used in some cases; however, it was necessary to design alternative methods for several TBI individuals. Justin had profound memory problems that resulted in his neglecting to use his diary or, alternatively, forgetting where he had put it. Hence, his choice of diary was a small notebook on a cord attached to a key ring that was hooked to his belt. Other TBI individuals were unable to remember the contents of a standard diary page once they closed their diaries. To overcome this problem, weekly planners were posted on a wall in the kitchen or in a bedroom. The planners thus served as diaries and provided a visual cue to record and recall information.

Following the selection of an appropriate type of diary, the TBI client and a family member were instructed in its use. Many participants had not been exposed to the diary system previously, and it was necessary to provide specific instructions regarding the type of information to be recorded, to state that it needed to be recorded as soon as it was heard or seen, and to devise a plan for the client to regularly check his or her diary. Retrieving information from diaries at each mealtime proved to be one effective strategy in this respect. There was a common misconception that diaries were to be used to record what had happened during the day, not to record information about future events. One client, Derek, took 2 months to learn to record future events and initially required repeated instructions regarding diary use from hospital staff and the therapist. Headings were made to help organize information in the diary. For example, one part of the diary page contained a "things to do" list, while another part contained an "appointments" list. The participant and therapist devised appropriate headings, the headings were explained several times, and the participant was requested to define them to a family member. A performance criterion for entry into the application phase was set whereby the TBI individual had to satisfactorily explain the diary system to the therapist on two separate occasions.

The application phase began with role plays in which the therapist would describe scenarios requiring diary use that occurred regularly in the participant's environment. The participant's task was to use the diary to record the information and then to explain to the therapist his plan for retrieving the information from the diary. Scenarios involved situations such as listing tasks assigned by an employer, taking phone messages, or recording tasks that needed to be completed around the house. When the participant was able to successfully use the diary in response to a range of scenarios, the therapist gave several pieces of information to the participant (e.g., "Your appointment is at 12:00 next week. Bring your diary with you, and bring your work assessment form"). A prompt was given to record this information in the diary, and the therapist also modeled performance by writing down the information in his or her diary. TBI clients were praised when they arrived for the next appointment at the correct time, with the correct equipment.

All rehabilitation team members utilized the same format, and team members prompted the individuals to check their diaries for the next day's activities. Family members were also encouraged to use a diary organization similar to that of the TBI individual's and to prompt the TBI individual to check his diary at the same time as they checked their own diaries. When participants were routinely using their diaries under these conditions, the verbal cues were slowly faded out. The therapist would prompt the individual only if he had not recorded appropriate information in his diary by the end of the session. Some participants had cognitive impairment so severe that they were not able to maintain diary use without prompts. In these cases, a series of visual prompts for diary use were devised, such as reminder notes on refrigerator doors. The use of visual prompts was found preferable for such individuals in that it reduces the degree of reliance on other people necessitated by verbal prompts.

The final phase, adaptation, involved assisting the TBI person to utilize the diary system in community settings. The primary task was to adapt the system so that the participant could easily and unobtrusively use a diary in any situation. Obtaining a diary of handier size, educating workmates to prompt the TBI individual to write down the information, and teaching the TBI individual to carry the diary at all times were frequently used interventions.

It was necessary that TBI individuals use the diary consistently for the diary to prove useful. At times, TBI individuals fluctuated between relying on their own memory and using the diary, with the result that neither strategy was successful. Inconsistent diary use was usually associated with changes in the degree of acceptance of impairment demonstrated by the TBI individuals. On the evidence of the improved performance that resulted from their diary use, several participants come to feel that their memory had somehow cured itself and ceased using their diaries. In such situations, the participants and their families were instructed to carry out an "experiment" in which they would use a diary for 1 week and would simply try to remember things for the next week. The performance during the two weeks would then be contrasted as a measure of the effectiveness of diary use.

Summary of the Procedure for Implementing Diary Use

1. Identify the type of information that the TBI individual needs to remember.
2. Choose a diary format best suited to the TBI individual's needs. For instance, some TBI individuals will need a dictaphone to record information; others will need the visual cues provided by a wall planner.
3. Inform the TBI individual that the diary needs to be available to him at all times and to be used consistently.
4. Reduce the possibility that the TBI individual will lose the diary by having the diary kept in a set place or by attaching the diary to the TBI individual (e.g., pocket diary attached to belt loop by a length of string).
5. Instruct the TBI individual as to the type of information to be recorded. In particular, stress that the diary is not a record of past events but is to operate as a method of recording information that needs to be remembered in the future.
6. Organize the diary so that information can be easily retrieved. This end can be achieved by dividing pages into headings such as "things to do," "phone calls to make," or "appointments."

7. Have the TBI individual explain the diary system that has been devised to the therapist and to a family member.
8. Inform the TBI individual that the information needs to be recorded in the diary as soon as it is given. Delays result in inaccurate recording or forgetting of the information.
9. Implement a plan for retrieval of information from the diary. Checking the diary at each mealtime is one effective strategy for information retrieval.
10. Describe scenarios to the TBI individual that require diary use. Have the TBI individual explain how he would record and retrieve the information given to him.
11. Set real-life tasks that require diary use for the TBI individual (e.g., give him a new appointment time). Give feedback on diary use. Praise him for successfully recording, retrieving, and acting upon the information.
12. Request that other health professionals and family members verbally prompt the TBI individual to use the diary system. Visual cues, such as notes reminding the TBI individual to use the diary, can also be effective in increasing diary use.
13. Monitor the TBI individual's use of the diary in community settings. Prompt the TBI individual to keep using the system and make any adaptations that are necessary for successful use (e.g., supplying a smaller or larger diary).

Environmental Compensation

Another external compensatory strategy employed was to alter the TBI client's physical environment to reduce the demands made upon memory. For example, the contents of Richard's cupboards were all clearly labeled so that he could locate ingredients without having to rely upon his memory. Similarly, Keith reorganized his workshop, placed all equipment into boxes that had the name of the equipment listed outside, and stored each box in a set place. The addition of notice boards, message pads near the telephone, and the strategy of leaving tools or materials out (e.g., on tables) as a reminder to complete a task also resulted in improved memory performance.

Checklists

When the information that TBI individuals forgot was related to a routine occurrence (e.g., a series of routine tasks), a system of checklists was devised. The checklists specified in written form the tasks that needed to be carried out and the order in which they were to be performed. When each task was completed, a check mark would be placed next to the appropriate item. A sample checklist is presented in Figure 3.1. This checklist was developed for Susan to ensure that she remembered to carry out certain jobs before leaving the house. Her husband frequently traveled on business and was therefore unable to prompt her or to check that tasks had been completed. The use of this checklist allowed her to independently complete the necessary tasks. Once a routine was firmly established in procedural memory, the use of the checklist was faded out. Initially, the checklist was used every second day, then once a week, and use was finally phased out once Susan was habitually completing the tasks. Procedural memory develops as the behavioral sequence contained in the checklist is learned through repeated learning trials and then finally becomes "automatic." When the sequence is established in procedural memory, the TBI individual will correctly implement the series of tasks, even though he or she may well be unable to recite the sequence.

Prompts

Prompts can be extremely valuable in cueing TBI individuals to remember information. Generalization of memory strategies can also be enhanced by placing prompts that remind TBI individuals to employ memory aids in different settings (McGlynn, 1990). As part of cognitive rehabilitation, both visual prompts (e.g., notes) and verbal prompts (e.g., spoken reminders from relatives) were utilized. For example, Justin found that when he woke up in the morning, he was disoriented for 10–15 minutes, during which time he had difficulty remembering what day it was, where he was, and what activities he needed to complete. A written note placed next to his bed each night successfully acted as a visual prompt to cue him regarding the day, date, and the first few activities of the day (e.g., showering and dressing). Objects in the physical environment also functioned as visual prompts. For example, Patrick wanted to remember to pay his bills on a regular basis. When a desk was placed in his living room with a clearly marked "bills" folder placed upon it, the frequency with which he paid his bills on time improved. Other visual prompts utilized included small stickers on refrigerators and cup-

Before leaving the house:	Check off when complete
1. Check that the elements on the stove are turned off.	☐
2. Check that all the lights are turned off.	☐
3. Put Joel's car seat in the car.	☐
4. Check that windows are closed; lock all doors.	☐
5. Put key in handbag.	☐
6. Fasten Joel's seat belt.	☐

FIGURE 3.1. Sample checklist.

board doors prompting diary use and notes left in strategic areas of the house (e.g., bedroom, bathroom).

As other researchers have found, verbal prompts are one of the most frequently employed memory aids adopted by TBI sufferers (see Wilson, 1992). Family members would often remind a TBI individual of the tasks he needed to carry out at the beginning of each day and in some cases would telephone the TBI individual to provide a further reminder nearer to the time a task needed to be completed. While this form of verbal prompting was very effective, families were advised, for a number of reasons, to use it circumspectly. First, verbal prompting requires the presence of a family member and is therefore available only when a family member is present. Second, extensive verbal prompting can lead to dependence on family members and reduce the incentive for the TBI individual to employ alternative memory strategies such as diary use. Third, verbal prompting by family members can lead to disharmony between the TBI individual and the family members if overutilized. For example, Grant encouraged his wife to verbally prompt him, only to later became angry with her "nagging" at him.

Other techniques have been described that could potentially be applied to increase the efficacy of verbal prompting. Sohlberg et al. (1992), for example, employ a strategy referred to as "prospective memory training" in which the TBI individual is given a prompt to carry out an activity at a future point in time (e.g., 2 minutes after the prompt). The length of time between when the prompt is given and the action is to be carried out is gradually increased as the TBI individual's performance improves. Case studies have been reported illustrating this memory-training technique, but as yet its efficacy has not been empirically evaluated.

Internal Compensatory Techniques

Mnemonic techniques are routinely taught as part of many cognitive rehabilitation programs. Strategies include semantic elaboration, in which the TBI individual determines what property objects to be remembered have in common; visual imagery, in which the TBI individual forms mental pictures of the information to be remembered; and verbal mediation, in which the TBI individual puts the words to be remembered into unusual sequences. These techniques are all encoding-level interventions and are thought to improve memory performance by providing a more elaborate memory trace that has associations with other information. Another frequently used internal compensatory strategy is the PQRST technique, which is designed to increase the recall of written information (Robinson, 1960). PQRST is an abbreviation for a five-step procedure that involves Previewing the text, developing Questions to ask after reading, Reading the text, Stating the answers to the questions, and Testing knowledge by checking the answer against the text. The PQRST method has good empirical support (Benedict, 1989).

Simple mnemonics techniques were routinely taught in the family support program as part of the education program. Strategies utilized included pairing a name with a characteristic feature of the individual (e.g., "curly-haired Kate") and visualizing the content of information as it was presented. With very specific problems, such as remembering the location of objects, these strategies worked well. However, the information that must be remembered in everyday life is very rarely in the form of discrete units such as paired associates or lists of words to be remembered (see also Zencius et al., 1991). Thus, in practice, the usefulness of mnemonics was restricted to a very limited range of situations. Difficulties were also encountered with TBI clients who did not have the necessary cognitive ability to learn the techniques, who had great difficulty trying to remember to use the techniques at appropriate times, and who felt that the techniques were peculiar. Because of these difficulties, the teaching of mnemonic strategies ceased during the first year of the program, and the program thereafter focused upon teaching the use of external memory aids. Other researchers have also noted that the use of mnemonics can be associated with limited generalization, too heavy a demand being placed upon the TBI individual's limited cognitive capacity, and compliance problems (e.g., McGlynn, 1990; O'Connor & Cermack, 1987; Sohlberg & Mateer, 1989).

Social Skills

One effective technique for coping with memory deficit proved to be teaching the TBI individuals how to communicate constructively with others about their memory impairment. When the TBI individuals gave some such explanation as "My memory isn't too good since the accident, so please remind me if I forget anything" to family members or employers in advance, tolerance and understanding were generally shown. If such explanations were not provided, memory lapses were frequently attributed to laziness or stupidity. Such attributions resulted in anger or frustration being directed toward the TBI individual. Therefore, the TBI persons were taught how to state clearly what their problem was, how it came about, and what the other person could do to help. To be effective, the statements needed to be kept brief and delivered in a somewhat humorous tone. Keith, for example, was concerned that he was repeating himself in conversations due to his poor short-term memory. He found it helpful to casually comment, "Did I just say that? I repeat myself sometimes since the accident. Just give me a nudge if I do it, okay?" This gave others the permission to give him feedback about the content of his conversation and greatly reduced his anxiety about his memory lapses.

Normalization and the Altering of Expectations

Following the TBI, some of the individuals and their families became sensitized to the presence of memory impairment and noted every memory lapse that occurred. Normalizing memory lapses by stating that everyone occasionally forgets information helped relieve some of the distress that the TBI sufferers felt in these situations. Reducing the saliency of memory lapses was important, as increased apprehension appeared to result in decreased recall and recognition on the part of many of the TBI individuals. High expectations regarding memory performance by either the individual or his family also resulted in increased apprehension and reduced memory performance. High expectations were particularly problematic for those individuals who had relied heavily upon their memory prior to injury. Educating families and employers that memory difficulties were common following TBI, and that expectations for performance needed to be reduced, assisted the TBI individuals to adjust their own expectations for performance. It was also necessary to inform families and employers that memory impairment did not necessarily imply reduced intelligence and that there were strategies that could help to improve the TBI individuals' performance.

COPING WITH ATTENTION PROBLEMS

Impairments of attention frequently result from TBI and are generally evident from the acute phase of injury onward. Unfortunately, there is a tendency for impairment of attention to be overlooked as a possible rehabilitation focus in favor of memory or perceptual impairment. Furthermore, some rehabilitation programs provide generalized cognitive rehabilitation without offering interventions targeted at attention as a separate function (Wood, 1988a). Rehabilitation emphasis on attention is increasing, however, due to recent findings indicating that computer-assisted retraining programs can produce some improvement on neuropsychological tests of attention (e.g., Ben-Yishay et al., 1987a; Sohlberg & Mateer, 1987; Rattok et al., 1992). Unfortunately, generalization of improvements on computer-training tasks to everyday tasks is limited, some studies finding that treatment effects do not spontaneously generalize to nontraining tasks (e.g., Niemann et al., 1990). Furthermore, other researchers have even found that once spontaneous recovery and practice effects are controlled for, there is little additional benefit due to intervention (Ponsford & Kinsella, 1988).

The approach taken in the family support program to the amelioration of attention deficits was to utilize compensatory techniques that could be broadly described as environmental management. Thus, participants were advised to alternate demanding cognitive tasks with more physical tasks. For instance, Patrick's ability to concentrate on administrative tasks (e.g., preparing invoices) improved markedly when this task was interspersed with gardening. Attention problems were also coped with by restricting the number of tasks carried out at any one time, thereby preventing division of attention between tasks. At work, Aaron found that he was unable to concentrate and was forgetting the instructions he had been given. Further analysis of the situation revealed that he was simultaneously carrying out three tasks at once. Restricting him to the completion of one task before moving on to the next resulted in his being able to complete each task successfully. Finally, participants were advised to ensure that they took adequate rest breaks, to avoid letting their gaze move around the room, and to reduce the amount of stimuli competing for attention (e.g., by not playing music while working).

PROCEDURES FOR ENHANCING NEW LEARNING

In contrast to the early recognition by TBI victims of their attention deficits, the severity of their learning difficulties often did not become apparent to them or their families for 8 months or more following injury. The reason for the delayed onset of recognition of learning difficulties appeared to be that opportunities for learning completely new information did not generally occur until many months after injury. Joseph and his parents, for example, maintained that he had no learning difficulties. However, when he attempted to obtain a truck driver's license, his learning difficulties became conspicuous. Changes in the physical environment, and the method of learning, helped increase the rate of new learning. For example, learning in quiet places away from distractions, note taking, studying in a set place, tackling small chunks of material at a time, and working for short periods of time (e.g., 10–15 minutes) were all useful strategies for improving learning of information (e.g., rote learning of road rules).

Some individuals had difficulty learning to use novel machinery and appliances (e.g., microwaves, new factory equipment). In these situations, a "guided practice" procedure was implemented. Guided practice involved a hands-on approach in which the procedure was first modeled by the "teacher." The "learner" then attempted the task while the "teacher" provided feedback and physical guidance if needed. Finally, the "learner" attempted the task independently using this procedure. Derek successfully learned basic cooking skills and how to use a new automatic washing machine using this method.

EXECUTIVE FUNCTIONING

According to Szekeres et al. (1987), the role of executive functioning is analogous to a manager whose task it is to set goals, plan and implement activity, monitor the performance of the system, initiate and inhibit behavior, and evaluate outcomes. Executive functioning has been attributed to the frontal area of the brain, which is known to be sensitive to damage from rotational forces that may cause the brain to impact the orbital ridges (Burke et al., 1991). Executive functioning is critical to TBI individuals' readjustment, in that it enables them to effectually regulate the basic cognitive skills that have remained intact following the injury. Having an intact memory, for example, will not greatly assist the TBI individual if he is unable to synthesize and formulate a plan from the information he has remembered.

Executive functioning may be impaired in a variety of ways. Motivational disturbances may prevent the TBI individual from perceiving a problem or attempting a solution. Limited creativity may result in the TBI individual's being unable to generate the possible options necessary to solve problems; alternatively, the TBI individual may be unable to isolate the essential components of information from those that are irrelevant (F. C. Goldstein & Levin, 1987). The three most frequently used strategies to cope with impaired executive functioning are described below.

Decision Making and Problem Solving

Because decision-making and problem-solving difficulties are so prevalent following TBI, the opportunity to make decisions needs to be given from the very early stages of recovery (Ylvisaker & Szekeres, 1989). Doing so encourages the development of reasoning and problem-solving skills, as well as provides an opportunity to give feedback on performance. Later on in the rehabilitation process, more structured interventions such as the D'Zurilla and Goldfried (1971) problem-solving technique can be employed. This technique was routinely utilized in the family support program in situations in which participants faced difficult decisions or problems. The technique was successfully applied to a wide range of situations such as deciding when to return to driving, when to leave high school, and whether or when to leave home to live in an apartment.

The problem-solving procedure was simplified when it was apparent that the TBI individuals' cognitive impairment made it problematic for them to use this quite complex multistep technique. For example, it was necessary to provide a handout for most TBI individuals with each stage of the problem-solving process noted down. The person then completed each step, recording the outcome as he proceeded. Carrying out the exercise jointly with the therapist using a white board to display the steps, and the conclusions reached at each step, was another effective modification. The utilization of the guided-practice strategy, in which the therapist modeled the procedure, then assisted the participant as he completed the procedure, and finally allowed the participant to complete the procedure independently, facilitated use of this technique.

It was important to provide TBI individuals with an opportunity to practice problem-solving skills. For example, Susan was having difficulty making decisions and was simply waiting passively for others to make them for her. Her refusal to make decisions was particularly obvious in occupational therapy sessions, in which she would sit in a chair until instructed by her occupational therapist in a step-by-step manner how to complete a task. Liaison with Susan's occupational therapist resulted in Susan's being given the opportunity to make numerous simple decisions during her therapy times (e.g., what colors she wanted to use as dyes) using the problem-solving method. This strategy resulted in an increase in Susan's decision-making attempts and an increase in the accuracy of her decision making.

A common obstacle to effective problem solving was that the TBI individual would attempt to solve a number of problems and make many decisions simultaneously. If TBI individuals displayed this tendency, they were taught to work on only the two most urgent decisions at any given time. Urgency was determined by whether the problem would have an immediate effect upon their safety (e.g., deciding about how to reduce their aggressive behavior), their basic survival needs (i.e., for food, shelter, and work), or their family (e.g., deciding whether to leave a partner). Once one problem had been successfully resolved, they would then move on to solving the problem of next greatest urgency.

Summary of the Problem-Solving Technique

Step 1. General orientation ("Stop and think").
Example: Don't get angry, stop and think about this.

Step 2. Problem definition and formulation ("What's the problem?").
Example: The problem is that my workshop supervisor is not happy with me.

Step 3. Information collection ("What information do I need?").
Example: I need to find out what, if anything, I did wrong. If I have done something wrong, I need to ask what I was supposed to do.

Step 4. Generation of alternatives ("What are possible solutions?").
Example: (a) I need to work more slowly.
(b) The task is too hard and I need to ask for a simpler, more routine task.
(c) I need to use some of the memory techniques I learned.

Step 5. Decision making ("Which is the best solution?").
Example: Well, my supervisor said that she told me to do a job three times and I still did not do it. Actually, I did not remember that she had told me. I need to use my memory techniques.

Step 6. Verification ("Did it work? Why?").
Example: Yes, it worked. When I wrote down the list of jobs, I could look back at the list and determine what to do next.

Planning Disorders

Task Analysis

One of the central elements of successful planning is the ability to accurately analyze a task and reduce it into its component parts. Participants in the family support program were frequently unable to do such task analysis. Derek reached a decision that he needed to structure his time more carefully, but reported that he had no idea how to do so. Similarly, Peter decided he wanted to move from home and live independently, but could not determine the necessary steps he needed to take in order to achieve his goal. To improve planning skills, TBI individuals were asked to select a basic task (e.g., weeding a garden, visiting a friend) and to write down the steps that were necessary to complete the task. If the TBI individual had difficulty with this procedure, the therapist would provide assistance. When a plan had been formulated, the TBI individual completed the tasks according to the steps he had generated. On completion of the task, the success or failure of the outcome was discussed with the therapist. The TBI individual then assessed the utility of the plan that had been made and wrote down any necessary adjustments to the steps he had previously decided upon. Ylvisaker and Szekeres (1989) have followed a similar process for improving planning ability by providing the TBI individual with a variety of imaginary scenarios (e.g., "What would you do if you lost your car keys?") and having him complete a series of questions designed to assist him to formulate an appropriate plan (e.g., "What is your goal?" "How can you . . . ?").

Self-Instructional Training

Self-instructional training (SIT) was originally developed by Meichenbaum, who used this technique to help impulsive children better control their behavior (Meichenbaum, 1977; Meichenbaum & Goodman, 1971). SIT involves a verbal mediation process in which the individual concerned initially talks out loud to himself throughout the task he is undertaking, then this "self-talk" becomes subvocal, and eventually verbal mediation becomes covert. Although originally used as a means of ameliorating attentional problems, SIT has been successfully applied to planning disorders and self-regulation problems following TBI (e.g., Cicerone & Wood, 1987; Craine, 1982). In the family support program, SIT was used to improve planning ability through a procedure in which the TBI individuals verbally coached themselves through the steps necessary to complete a task. In addition to verbalizing the necessary steps, the TBI individuals also asked questions out loud, such as, "What materials do I need?" or "How long do I have to complete this?" In some cases, the steps needed to complete a task were written down because of the TBI individual's memory impairment. The TBI individual then referred to the written instructions and read them aloud as he was completing the tasks. In practice, the covert phase, during which it was hoped that the TBI individual would be able to mentally coach himself through the task, was seldom reached. Hence, many of the TBI individuals who chose to utilize SIT continued to "mutter" to themselves when planning and implementing novel tasks.

Checklists

When TBI individuals demonstrated a persistent inability to formulate and implement plans, checklists were used. A good example of this was a checklist developed for Derek by a roommate. When it was Derek's turn to shop for groceries, he repeatedly had difficulties planning a method to enable him to successfully complete this task. He frequently overspent and bought large quantities of certain items, while forgetting to purchase others. To overcome these problems, his roommate compiled a checklist of the necessary steps (e.g., check the cupboards, determine how much money was available). In addition, he made a comprehensive list of grocery items, arranged by food groups, with quantities and brands specified (Figure 3.2). Derek checked off the items that were not in the cupboard and made a second check mark when he had purchased them. The order

Item	Not in cupboard	Bought?
Fruit		
5 apples	☐	☐
4 pears	☐	☐
12 bananas	☐	☐
Vegetables		
1 cabbage	☐	☐
Hoyts potatoes, 2 kg bag	☐	☐
Carrots, 7 medium, not in bag	☐	☐
Barkers onions, 1.5 kg bag	☐	☐
Dairy food		
Guaranted basics:		
Colby cheese, 1 kg	☐	☐
Pam's standard milk, 2 liters	☐	☐
Country soft blend margarine, 500 g	☐	☐
Laundry products		
Drive laundry powder, 1.5 kg	☐	☐
Sunlight dishwashing liquid, 900 ml	☐	☐
Hygenix 1-ply toilet roll, package of 4	☐	☐
Frend stain remover, 350 ml can	☐	☐

FIGURE 3.2. Sample shopping list.

of the items on the grocery list was the same as the order in which the items were arranged in the local supermarket. This method was extremely effective and allowed Derek to continue to carry out his household management responsibilities.

GENERALIZATION

An ongoing rehabilitation concern is whether the skills learned will transfer from the training setting into the community setting and thereby result in functional gains. Researchers have found that TBI individuals do not automatically transfer skills from a learning task to more functional activities or from setting to setting (Benedict, 1989; Szekeres et al., 1987). It has been hypothesized that this lack of generalization may be related to frontal lobe dysfunction that has reduced abstract reasoning ability (Niemann et al., 1990). Regardless of causation, if generalization is to occur, the intervention program must include specific strategies to enhance generalization (Gordon & Hibbard, 1992).

As part of the cognitive compensatory intervention, a number of strategies aimed at improving generalization were employed. The cognitive compensation skills were always taught in the context of everyday situations (e.g., teaching diary use by making "to be remembered" appointment times). Skills were repeatedly practiced until their use was largely automatic, the skills were taught in a variety of settings (e.g., in the home, in the workplace) by a variety of different people (e.g., the occupational therapist, work tutor, psychologist), and visual and verbal prompts to cue strategy use were devised (e.g., a note on the bathroom mirror, or a family member reminding the TBI individual to take her diary). When participants demonstrated that they had generalized skills across settings, verbal praise was given. While these prompting strategies had some degree of success, it was apparent that those individuals with more severe executive dysfunction required continual prompting to use the compensation strategies.

Summary of the Procedure for Facilitating Generalization

1. Teach strategies in the context of everyday situations.
2. Encourage the TBI individual to repeatedly practice the strategy, until the use of the strategy is largely automatic.
3. Teach strategies in a variety of different settings.
4. Arrange for several different people to teach the same strategy.
5. Provide visual and verbal prompts to cue the use of the strategy.
6. Provide verbal praise when the TBI individual utilizes the strategies.

FAMILY INVOLVEMENT IN COGNITIVE REHABILITATION

With the agreement of the TBI individual, the family was invited to attend sessions that addressed cognitive compensation. The family was in the unique position of being able to monitor the TBI individual's progress, prompt the TBI individual to use the compensatory strategies, and rehearse the compensatory skills with the TBI individual on a daily basis. However, in order for the family to be able to assist the TBI individual, it was necessary to provide education about the strategies, to supply written instructions about what could be done to assist the TBI individual, and to plan with the family the pragmatics of how they could implement the strategies. The demands that could reasonably be made upon a family varied according to the time available to them and their financial and personal resources. Overburdening a family could lead to anger or feelings of failure when they could not cope. Finally, it was critical to encourage the family to have realistic expectations of the TBI individual's performance that matched the therapist's expectations. If similar expectations were not held, then the demands made upon the TBI individual by the family would be either excessive (e.g., request 2 hours of PQRST practice daily) or very limited (e.g., tell him not to bother using a diary).

Families reported that from their perspective, the most useful intervention was a "troubleshooting" exercise in which the therapist role played a variety of problematic scenarios (e.g., the TBI individual's refusing to use a diary or becoming angry when reminded to take a shower). The therapist, the TBI individual, and the family then discussed the possible options for dealing with the scenario, such as using distraction techniques, offering social reinforcement for compliance, or giving the individual more time to complete the task. When the family expressed discomfort at discussing potential problems in front of the TBI individual, a separate appointment was made to discuss the issues without the person present. Throughout the support program, both the TBI individual and the family could request separate sessions, although joint sessions were more frequently used.

IMPLEMENTING COGNITIVE COMPENSATORY STRATEGIES

Most compensatory strategies are not conceptually complex. However, clinical experience has indicated that the successful implementation of compensatory strategies requires considerable skill on the therapist's part. As noted earlier, careful assessment is crucial if the primary problem underlying the deficit in performance is to be accurately identified. It is also essential to incorporate the clients' input into the choice of intervention strategy. Failure to do so may result in noncompliance (see also Kreutzer et al., 1989). Some compensatory strategies were quite foreign to the TBI individuals' preinjury way of life (e.g., a factory worker who associated diaries with corporate businesspeople). Other TBI individuals stated that the degree of cognitive impairment they experienced did not warrant the effort required to implement the compensatory strategies. It was quite common for the TBI individual to find the cognitive compensatory strategy unacceptable for some reason (e.g., it required too much effort to use), to devalue its worth, and finally to discontinue using it. Accordingly, comprehensive education about cognitive impairment and the purpose of compensatory techniques was provided. All techniques were then introduced as "suggestions," and only after detailed discussion would mutually agreed-upon cognitive compensatory strategies be chosen. Introducing one strategy at a time was preferable, as it avoided overwhelming the TBI individuals and their families. This was particularly important for TBI individuals who were having difficulty adjusting in several domains (e.g., socially, vocationally, emotionally) and were struggling to cope.

In addition to involving clients in the choice of strategies, the implementation of strategies was monitored, feedback was provided, and praise was given for consistent strategy use. This process is important, as the TBI individual's skills and needs change over time (Kreutzer et al., 1989). When necessary (e.g., for problem-solving strategies), direct assistance was provided to the TBI individual; however, this assistance was later gradually faded out. Another helpful implementation technique was to build upon the TBI individual's preexisting compensatory strategies. For example, when neuropsychological testing was carried out, it became obvious that Aaron was performing better than would be expected given the severity of his injury. Questioning revealed that even before the accident, he had used visual imagery to enhance his recall. Tailoring his use of visual imagery provided him with an effective technique that had heuristic value for him.

Finally, it was necessary to recognize the interaction between cognitive compensation and psychosocial functioning. Each TBI individual and his family presented with a unique psychosocial profile of educational experiences, motivation, awareness of deficit, interpersonal skills, and emotional state. Consequently, interventions were tailored to meet the TBI individual's specific needs. For example, with some TBI individuals, it was necessary to teach skills very gradually in order to prevent the failure they desperately feared. In contrast, other TBI individuals became frustrated with this approach and requested that they learn a number of strategies that they could then "experiment with" to determine which strategies were most effective.

Summary of the Procedure for Facilitating Cognitive Strategies Implementation

1. Assess the TBI individual's cognitive functioning carefully to help identify the primary problem underlying the performance impairment.

2. Select compensatory strategies in collaboration with the TBI individual and his family.
3. Enhance preexisting compensatory strategies before teaching novel techniques.
4. Select strategies that place the least demands upon the TBI individual and that have face validity for him.
5. Provide comprehensive education about cognitive impairment and the purpose of compensatory strategies.
6. Introduce only one or two strategies at any given time.
7. Introduce strategies as "suggestions." Tell the TBI individual and the family that the strategy will be tried to see if it is helpful and to see if modifications are needed to ensure that it is useful.
8. Monitor the implementation of all strategies, provide feedback on the TBI individual's use of the strategy, and give praise when strategies are used consistently and appropriately.
9. Tailor compensatory strategies to take account of the TBI individual's overall presentation (e.g., emotional state, level of motivation, support available from family).

COMPENSATING FOR COGNITIVE IMPAIRMENT: AN ILLUSTRATIVE CASE STUDY

Brian was a 17-year-old male who had sustained a TBI in a motorcycle accident immediately before he was to commence a new position as an apprentice mechanic. He had a posttraumatic amnesia of 5 days, and neuropsychological assessment 6 months after injury revealed short- and long-term verbal memory deficits on the Russell Revision of the Wechsler Memory Scale (E. W. Russell, 1975). His scores on the Paced Auditory Serial-Addition Task (Gronwall, 1977) were also indicative of slowed information processing. His father, with whom he was living, noted that he was more frequently withdrawn, moody, and unmotivated than before the accident. Brian himself was not aware of these changes and went to work almost immediately after being discharged from the hospital. However, when his employer was contacted some months later to assess his progress, several concerns were raised. His employer stated that Brian was "not with it"; he was forgetting to do tasks and failing to remember to carry out routine safety checks. An incident had occurred in which a vehicle had almost left the workshop with loose wheel nuts. The safety implications of this incident troubled his employer greatly.

With Brian's agreement, for a 1-week period the employer recorded all incidents in which Brian forgot to complete aspects of work tasks. This information was used to design an appropriate intervention strategy. A combination of a notebook and checklists was chosen by Brian. All jobs given were immediately written in the notebook, and Brian would read back the entry to whoever assigned the task in order to ensure that he had noted it down correctly. Once the job was completed, it was crossed off the page. The checklists contained the safety tasks that needed to be carried out (e.g., removing mats from the car before beginning welding). Safety tasks were also checked off the list when they had been completed. The therapist monitored the system by questioning Brian, in order to ensure that Brian found it useful and was continuing to employ it. Five weeks after the implementation of the program, Brian reported that he was now carrying out all safety checks routinely without needing the checklist. He had continued to use the notebook, as he found it very helpful. When his employer was contacted again, he reported that he was no longer noticing any memory-related problems in the work setting.

4

Enhancing Emotional Adjustment

Many individuals with traumatic brain injury (TBI) and their family members experience some form of adverse emotional reaction such as anxiety, depression, grief, or low self-esteem following the injury (Brooks et al., 1986; Tyerman & Humphrey, 1984). These adverse emotional reactions are not surprising, given the large number of adjustments that TBI individuals and their families face. This chapter describes the approach taken in the family support program to enhance emotional adjustment following TBI. The interventions employed in the program are primarily based on the Prigatano (1987a) model, in which reactive responses (e.g., depression, irritability), neuropsychological factors (e.g., impulsivity), and long-standing characterological styles (e.g., dependency) are all seen to impact upon the TBI individual's personality and emotional functioning. According to Prigatano's model, the choice of intervention is then guided by whether the problem is primarily reactionary, neuropsychological, or characterological. For instance, reactionary-type adverse emotional reactions are addressed within a psychotherapeutic mode, rather than being treated with psychotropic medication. Similarly, neuropsychological problems are managed using environmental modification or cognitive coping strategies, rather than psychotherapy (Prigatano, 1986).

The Lazarus and Folkman (1984) stress-appraisal and coping model was also utilized to guide the development of the intervention approach for emotional problems. According to this model, stress occurs when the person experiences environmental demands that exceed his or her ability to cope. In the case of TBI, it is hypothesized that as individuals discover that they are no longer able to cope with the demands placed upon them, adverse emotional reactions result. These adverse reactions can be ameliorated by altering mediating variables such as coping skills, appraisal, and social support. Godfrey, Knight, and Partridge (1994) provide a discussion of this model applied to emotional adjustment following TBI.

MANAGING DEPRESSION

The estimated prevalence of clinical depression in TBI victims varies from 27% to 60% (e.g., Brooks et al., 1986; Elsass & Kinsella, 1987; Kinsella et al., 1988; Tyerman & Humphrey, 1984). Depression appears to be reactive in nature and is associated with losses sustained after the injury (e.g., failing to return to work, personality change) and decreased self-esteem (Godfrey et al., 1994). As TBI individuals' awareness of their impairments increases, their depressive symptomatology also increases (Boake, Freeland, Reinghalz, Nance, & Edwards, 1987). Similarly, as families acknowledge the permanent changes evidenced by TBI individuals, they may become quite dysphoric. The risk of suicide by TBI individuals can be high, not only because of the increased rates of depression following TBI, but also because the majority of TBI individuals are already in a high-risk category, being male and under 25 and having low socioeconomic status (Shaffer, Garland, Gould, Gisher, & Trautman, 1988). Furthermore, the poor impulse control associated with TBI increases the risk that suicidal ideation will be acted upon. Support, monitoring, and intervention for depression are therefore especially important for TBI individuals.

Cognitive Strategies

One of the characteristic features of depression is persistent negative ruminations that are thought to worsen mood (Fennell, 1989). Peter, for example, spent much of his day thinking thoughts such as "I'll kill myself if I stay like this" and "Work tomorrow will probably be too much." The presence of negative thinking and consequent depression in TBI individuals has also been documented by other researchers (e.g., Malec, 1984). In the family support program, the TBI individuals and their families were encouraged to identify their negative thoughts and then replace them with more positive thoughts. This process was initially carried out in writing with therapist assistance. With practice, most family members and some of the higher-functioning TBI individuals were able to identify and replace thoughts independently. The TBI individuals were given a small card that contained some of the depressive statements that they habitually thought, the injunction STOP THINKING THIS written in capital letters underneath these statements, and a positive replacement statement written at the bottom of the card. The TBI individual then referred to the card at mealtimes each day or when he recognized that he was thinking negatively. All replacement statements were designed to be positive and realistic. At no time were TBI individuals or their families encouraged to use replacement statements such as "I'm feeling better than ever before" or "I can achieve anything I want to." Such statements tend to exacerbate problems with lack of awareness and denial of deficits. A sample "rethinking" card is illustrated in Figure 4.1.

In order to further reduce the amount of time TBI individuals and families

> "I'll never be able to do this. I'm useless."
>
> STOP THINKING THIS
>
> "Yes, I'm a bit slower now, but if I keep going step by step, I know I can do this."

FIGURE 4.1. Sample "rethinking card."

spent in negative rumination, they were encouraged to distract themselves by engaging in an alternative activity or by using thought-stopping techniques. Graham's thought-stopping strategy, for instance, was to imagine a lightning bolt going through his brain and simultaneously to say aloud, "Stop thinking." Both the thought-stopping and distraction techniques were extremely effective. Figure 4.2 displays the decrease in Graham's episodes of suicidal thinking after he began replacing negative thoughts and utilizing distraction and thought-stopping strategies.

Behavioral Strategies

Activity Scheduling

Following traumatic brain injury, victims are often no longer able to participate in a number of activities that were highly enjoyable to them prior to the injury (e.g., motorcycle riding). This inability results in decreased participation in pleas-

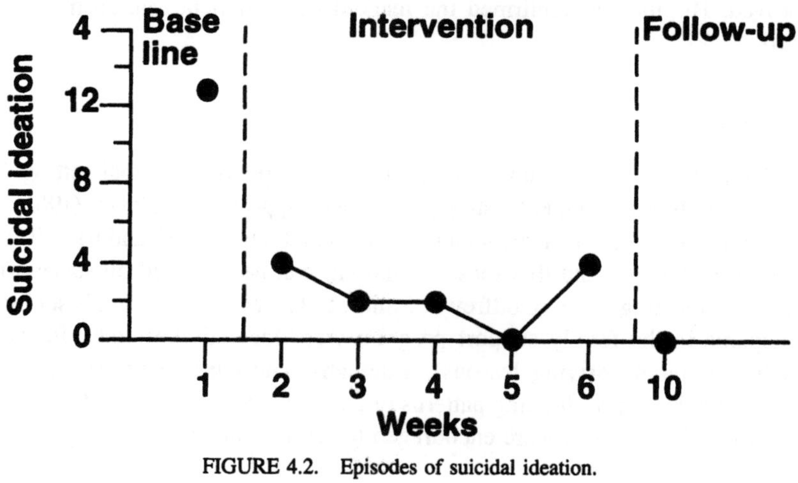

FIGURE 4.2. Episodes of suicidal ideation.

ant events and increased negative thinking (Lewinsohn, Munoz, Youngren, & Zeiss, 1986). Hence, to counter depression, an important intervention strategy is to schedule alternative rewarding activities (Godfrey & Smith, 1992). Activity scheduling was carried out with all depressed TBI individuals. A graded approach was employed involving setting small achievable steps first, with more difficult activities being scheduled by the therapist once the smaller goals had been achieved. Peter, for example, initially spent time completing a simple scheduled activity with his sister (e.g., watching a video, going out for a meal). Four weeks later, he joined a volleyball team and then began inviting friends to his house for a meal. These activities were chosen because they were intrinsically reinforcing, prevented negative rumination, and provided opportunities for social reinforcement. Exercise was an activity that was found to be particularly effective in reducing depression. For example, both Grant and his wife noted that his mood improved when he ran regularly.

The effect of participation in reinforcing activities on mood was dramatic in some cases. For instance, Justin's mood had been stable for several months and he was receiving only case-monitoring sessions at 6-week intervals. However, 5 weeks after a follow-up visit, he became severely depressed. At this time, he reported significant levels of suicidal ideation, headaches, and disrupted sleep. On two occasions, he had felt that he had heard voices talking to him about concepts of time travel. During the 5 weeks between follow-up visits, he quit his part-time job, moved back to his parents' house, and was spending much of his time lying in bed. His days were lacking in structure, and he was engaging in few, if any, pleasant activities. After careful assessment, Justin and the therapist agreed that it appeared that lack of reinforcing activity had led to his sudden depressed mood. Justin was then advised to attend a full-time course at a local college. He greatly enjoyed the college course, and within a month his sleep returned to normal, his headaches disappeared, he stopped hearing voices, and his mood and self-esteem improved. His mother confirmed the marked improvement that Justin had reported.

Goal Setting

Another important behavioral treatment for depression is goal setting. The setting of goals as a therapeutic strategy was first suggested by Glasser (1965). For the TBI individual, the achievement of personal mastery (Bandura, 1977) is central to happiness, and this sense of mastery can be achieved by successfully setting and meeting goals (Godfrey & Smith, 1992). Most of the goals set by the participants in the family support program were for activities (e.g., for social activities or taking driving lessons), although some participants set goals for changes in behavior or thinking patterns (e.g., to reduce the amount of time spent ruminating). Participants were encouraged to set a limited number of goals (i.e., no more than three), which were written down, quantifiable, and could be achieved within two weeks. Goals that required more than two weeks to complete were often found to be too complex, and in many cases the TBI individual would not have possessed the necessary skills to complete the task. All time limits for the completion of goals were flexible, as it was not always possible to anticipate delays such as illness or medical appointments. If either the TBI individual or his family were to have interpreted the time limits as unalterable, the late completion of a goal would have been considered a failure, precipitating further depression.

For the TBI individuals who had motivation difficulties, positive and negative contingencies were put in place when goals were consistently not achieved. These negative consequences were mild but very effective. For example, Richard forfeited the right to wear his favorite hat for a set period of time if he had met none of his goals during a week. This contingency greatly increased the number of goals he successfully met. Having a family member or friend prompt the TBI individual about the goals, and the progress that had been made, also improved motivation. If friends or family were unable to prompt the TBI individual, the therapist would telephone at the midpoint between sessions and question the TBI individual regarding his progress.

When the TBI individual or family member did not complete a goal, the reasons for this failure were discussed, and a problem-solving exercise was employed. Failure was generally attributed to the therapist's and the participant's having both neglected to adequately follow the goal-setting procedure (e.g., "We did not think about the fact that you have little money" or "We forgot that you are only in the early phases of recovery and still feel too tired to go running"). This prevented the participant's attributing the failure to an internal characteristic (e.g., "I'm dumb"), which would further exacerbate depression. Failure to complete goals provided the therapist with an excellent opportunity to model a positive approach to coping with this very common occurrence.

When the goals were successfully completed, the therapist complimented the participant for the achievement. Self-reinforcement, through verbalization of affirming statements, was also encouraged when goals were achieved. Both the TBI individuals and their families appeared to find the positive experience of setting and attaining goals a helpful strategy for improving mood. Goal setting also served to help participants learn new skills and increase their productivity. Other authors have noted similar improvements with the use of goal setting with TBI individuals (e.g., Gobble et al., 1987).

Summary of the Procedure for Goal Setting

Step 1. Client and therapist meet together and discuss goals.
Step 2. No more than three goals are chosen.

Step 3. Goals are written down in behavioral terms.
Example: To go swimming three times. To visit Aunt Margaret at her home on one occasion.

Step 4. A time limit is set within which goals are to be completed.
Example: One week.

Step 5. Goals are checked to ensure that they are realistic.
Example: Does Peter have the skills to carry out these two goals? Yes.

Step 6. Any foreseeable difficulties that may arise in meeting the goals are discussed.
Example: Is transport available? Does Peter know how to purchase tickets at the swimming pool? What if Peter decides tomorrow that he no longer wants to go swimming?

Step 7. A method of prompting the TBI individual to remember to complete the goals is devised.
Example: Peter's friend Dave will call him on Tuesday to check whether Peter has gone swimming yet.

Step 8. Contingencies are put in place.
Example: If both goals are completed within the week, Peter will buy himself a new music cassette.

Step 9. Progress toward goals is monitored and verbally reinforced by each session.
Example: At the next session, the therapist asks, "How did you get on with your goals this week?"

Step 10. If goals are not successfully completed, a problem-solving exercise is undertaken. If the goal was unrealistic, then this circumstance is acknowledged, and a new, more achievable goal is set.
Example: Therapist and participant identify the factors that led to the failure to meet the goal and then formulate a plan to rectify the problems.

Step 11. New goals are set when previous goals have been successfully completed.

Preventative Strategies

One of the principal methods used to prevent depression was to undermine the assumptions on which depressive thinking is based (Fennell, 1989). The most frequent underlying assumption made by the TBI victims was that in order to be happy, they *needed to be able to perform as well as they had performed prior to their accidents.* This assumption led them to make repeated attempts to carry out tasks that were no longer within their capability. Naturally, task failure was commonly associated with depressive thinking. The same process occurred with family members who expected that the TBI individual would be able to perform at his or her preinjury level. When this expectation was repeatedly dashed, depression resulted.

Helping the TBI individuals and families change their performance expectations presented a major challenge, yet it was essential to do so if depression was to be prevented. Modified rational emotive therapy techniques (A. Ellis, 1962) were employed to help participants test their underlying assumptions regarding their performance. Peter, for example, was challenged to think about whether a person with a broken leg should expect to run a marathon and then consider himself a failure when he found that he was unable to do so. Other TBI individuals role played situations in which the position was reversed, and they had to advise a close friend who had a traumatic brain injury and was expecting too much of himself.

In some cases, the TBI client or family member was given an assignment to test his or her underlying assumption in real life. Graham firmly believed that his workmates liked him only when he worked hard. One week working long hours, as compared to one week working normal hours, resulted in no changes in his workmates' attitudes toward him. In fact, they preferred him to work shorter hours, as he worked better when he was less tired. The analogy was made that having high expectations is like climbing a mountain: The higher the mountain, the farther the fall and the longer it takes to climb up again. Similarly, the higher the expectations, the greater the failure and depression and the longer it takes to readjust afterward.

Reattribution of causation from an internal locus (e.g., "I'm useless") to an external locus (e.g., "The task is difficult") (Weiner, Heckhausen, & Meyer, 1972) proved to be another important preventative technique. Derek, for instance, became depressed if he interpreted his motor slowness at occupational therapy tasks as a sign of his permanent inability to carry out tasks. However, if he correctly attributed his motor slowness to the early phase of his physical recovery and his high levels of fatigue, then his mood improved. The final preventative technique was to help TBI individuals make practical changes in some of the problem areas that led to depression. For example, Joseph's mood improved when he began special exercises to correct the droop in his shoulder that he felt made him look ugly.

MANAGING ANXIETY

There are very few references in the TBI rehabilitation literature to the treatment of anxiety disorders that may develop following brain injury. Some TBI participants in the program did develop anxiety disorders, although anxiety disorders occurred with significantly less frequency than did depressive reactions. These anxiety disorders tended to be either simple or social phobias, rather than generalized anxiety states. The most common simple phobia was fear of driving. Some TBI individuals also displayed performance anxiety related to specific situations (e.g., returning to work, using computers), and some family members became extremely anxious about the TBI individual's health or the possibility of further accidents occurring to themselves or others. Five main techniques were used to assist TBI individuals and their families to manage their anxiety. These techniques were based upon cognitive behavioral interventions for anxiety described by Beck and Emery (1985).

Relaxation Training

An abbreviated form of progressive muscle relaxation (Wolpe & Lazarus, 1966) was taped and given to participants who reported feeling tension in their muscles or feeling agitated and fidgety. The relaxation exercises were initially carried out with the therapist present. Once the TBI individuals or family members felt comfortable with the exercises, they then practiced them on a regular basis in their homes using a tape-recorded version of the progressive muscle-relaxation exercises. In addition to progressive muscle relaxation, the TBI individuals or family members learned breathing control techniques (i.e., how to breathe slowly and regularly) and in vivo relaxation. Unfortunately, the progressive muscle-relaxation training tended to be met with low compliance, as the participants reported that they found it inconvenient to carry out the exercises on a regular basis. The in vivo protocol, which involved tensing and relaxing various muscles during the course of daily activities, was more readily utilized by the participants. Other researchers have also used relaxation training with TBI individuals (autogenic relaxation, breathing exercises, and biofeedback) with some success (e.g., Lysaght & Bodenhamer, 1990).

Scheduling Relaxing Activities

The scheduling of relaxing activities was found to be more effective than the structured relaxation training in ameliorating anxiety problems. In scheduling relaxing activities, the TBI individual or family member drew up a list of calming activities (e.g., sitting in a quiet place, taking a bath). These activities were then allocated a time in the participant's daily planner. Ongoing monitoring was carried out by the therapist to ensure that the TBI individual or family member was completing the scheduled activities.

Graduated Exposure

Anxiety often leads to the avoidance of feared situations. Peter, for example, failed to attend computer classes because he feared he would not be able to learn how to use the computers, and Richard refused to drive because he feared he was a "jinx" and would cause another accident. Graduated exposure was the principal intervention strategy used to deal with such anxieties. Graduated exposure involves systematically exposing the person to the avoided stimuli in a graduated manner that does not elicit overwhelming emotional reactions (Wolpe, 1961). With repeated exposure to the anxiety-provoking stimuli, the person habituates to anxiety and relearns more adaptive responses. Peter's fear of computer classes was ameliorated in this manner. Initially, he began to learn about computers alongside an occupational therapist who later left him to work on the computers alone. Eventually, he attended the computer classes with extra tutoring, which was then faded out across an 8-week period. Other TBI individuals required repeated exposure to a single situation before anxiety reduced. For example, Patrick's anxiety regarding mistakes at work was alleviated only after he was instructed to repeatedly make mistakes. After 2 months, he acknowledged that making mistakes did not have the disastrous consequences that he had feared, and his work-related performance anxiety abated.

Cognitive Strategies

A variety of cognitive distortions, such as misinterpretation of events and hypervigilance, have been found to characterize anxiety disorders (Butler, 1989). Given the predominance of cognitive factors in anxiety disorders, an important focus of intervention for the participants' anxiety was teaching them to reinterpret situations and symptoms in a less threatening manner. For example, Justin concluded that he was going blind on the basis of the blurred vision that resulted from headache pain, and Richard's fear that he was a "jinx" and caused accidents stemmed from his having been in three car accidents in the previous two years. When misinterpretation occurred, participants were encouraged to reinterpret anxiety-provoking events by writing down the anxiety-provoking thoughts and then generating and writing down alternative, less anxiety-provoking thoughts. For some TBI individuals, this was too complex a task, and distraction techniques were employed as a simpler alternative coping strategy. Justin, for instance, focused on external features in a room (e.g., count the books on a bookshelf) when he began to ruminate about going blind. This stratagem proved to be a very effective anxiety-reduction technique for him. Butler (1989) provides a more detailed description of the use of cognitive strategies in the reduction of anxiety.

Risk Minimization

For many TBI individuals, the anxiety they experienced reflected realistic concerns. The objective risk of failure in social and vocational settings is greater following TBI. Likewise, the consequences of a second traumatic brain injury are likely to be worse than the consequences of the first brain injury. Fears that reflected realistic concerns required a "risk-minimization strategy." Risk minimization involved helping the TBI individual or family use a problem-solving format to analyze risk situations and identify the strategies they could use to reduce the risk. The risk-minimization strategies involved changes in their behavior (e.g., refusing to travel with drunk friends) or in their environment (e.g., obtaining a white board to write down information) or learning new skills (e.g., learning extra work-related skills). The use of such strategies appeared to result in reduced anxiety as TBI individuals gained a sense of control (Bandura, 1977) over the situations they had previously feared.

Managing Anxiety: An Illustrative Case Study

Prior to his TBI, Graham had been self-employed in a business in which he invested most of his time and energy. He was single, participated in very few social activities, and was prone to periods of severe depression. He had not, however, received any formal treatment for depression. In 1991, he sustained a TBI in a sporting accident. The exact nature of the injury was unclear, but was thought to involve a combination of anoxia and traumatic injury resulting in diffuse damage. His period of posttraumatic amnesia was 10 days. Following the TBI, Graham became highly anxious about both his ability to perform at work and his ability to socialize with other people (particularly females). He was experiencing what he termed "nervous episodes," during which his thoughts would race and he would sweat and feel nauseous. These episodes occurred on a daily basis, either at work or when he was in social settings. One year after the accident, his score on the Hamilton Anxiety Rating Scale (Hamilton, 1959), a clinician rating scale, was high (x = 17) and his State–Trait Anxiety Inventory (STAI) scores (Spielberger, Gorsuch, Lushene, Vagg, & Jacobs, 1983) were at the 92nd percentile for current anxiety and 97th percentile for general anxiety. Daily ratings of the number of nervous episodes he experienced indicated that approximately three occurred each week. This number was probably an underestimation, as Graham had been avoiding the situations that precipitated the nervous episodes (e.g., visiting others).

The use of progressive muscle relaxation alone proved ineffective for Graham. However, a combination of exposure and cognitive restructuring proved more efficacious. Each day, Graham wrote down his anxiety-provoking thoughts, along with alternative, more helpful ways of thinking. Role plays were used to help him reappraise anxiety-provoking situations. For instance, Graham felt anxious at work because of his belief that any mistake he made meant that he was a failure as a person. To reappraise this belief, Graham was asked to participate in a role play in which he had to comfort a friend at work who felt a failure because he had made a mistake. The statements Graham used to comfort his friend (e.g., "Every-

one makes mistakes") were then utilized to help Graham challenge his own belief that making mistakes equated with failure as a person. Attention was also paid to help him form realistic expectations about his performance in social settings. For instance, his belief that he should be able to make at least three new friends at a given social event (e.g., a wedding) had resulted in severe anxiety when he not surprisingly failed to do so. Finally, goals were set each week for him to expose himself to feared situations (e.g., inviting a neighbor over to tea).

Reassessment, 1 month after intervention began, revealed a significant reduction in the number of nervous episodes (see Figure 4.3) and a drop in his score on the Hamilton Rating Scale to 12. His self-report STAI scores, however, remained unchanged. A 6-week follow-up assessment documented a further drop in the Hamilton Rating Scale score to 7, and a maintenance of the decrease in nervous episodes. However, the STAI scores again remained high even though Graham himself reported that he felt much more relaxed and that he "hardly even noticed" the nervousness episodes.

THE GRIEVING PROCESS: ACCEPTING LOSS

An important psychological prerequisite to emotional adjustment following TBI is accepting the "losses" that follow TBI (Godfrey & Smith, 1992). Examples of losses include impaired abilities (e.g., cognitive functioning), decreased satisfaction with relationships, inability to drive, and failure to resume preinjury vocational status. TBI victims and their families grieve not only for the loss of prior abilities but also for the abilities that they thought would develop in the

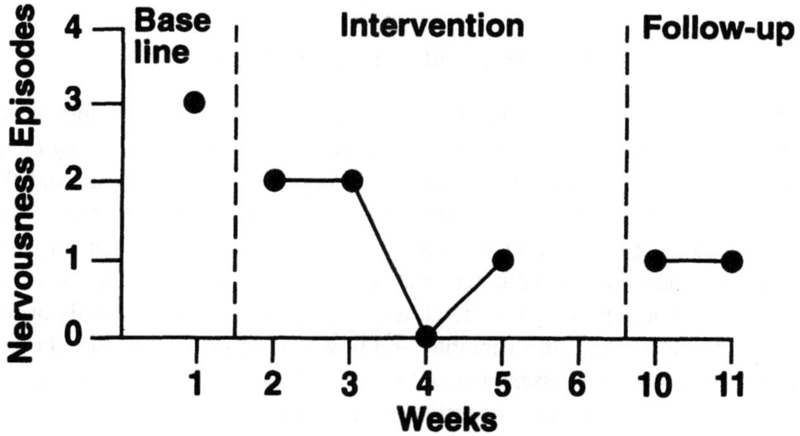

FIGURE 4.3. Frequency of nervousness episodes.

future (Gordon & Hibbard, 1992). Unfortunately, there is little published literature regarding grief following TBI. In the sparse existent literature, acceptance of loss is conceptualized either as a grief process or as a process of acceptance. For example, Muir and Haffey (1984), as noted in Chapter 2, refer to accepting loss as the "mobile mourning process," while Prigatano and Fordyce (1986b) and Ben-Yishay et al. (1985) refer to the process as one of "acceptance" whereby TBI individuals and their families concede that some functions cannot be further improved upon.

The grief process following TBI does stand in contrast to many other grief processes (e.g., the death of a partner, redundancy) in that it involves uncertainty. Over the first year following injury, it can be extremely difficult to identify those functions that are permanently damaged and hence require "acceptance of loss" and those functions that may recover or be adequately compensated for. For example, the process of determining whether a TBI sufferer will be able to return to work can be lengthy. Throughout this process, both the TBI individual and his family may fluctuate between acceptance of loss and despair depending on whether they perceive the problem of employability to be resolvable or not. According to Muir and Haffey (1984), the uncertainty in the loss process results in four characteristic features of TBI-related grief: (1) The grief process will include a search for the certainty of recovery; (2) the TBI individual and his family will fluctuate between euphoria and despair; (3) feelings of rage will be exacerbated; and (4) the uncertainty can result in learned helplessness. Muir and Haffey (1984) state that these features can be counteracted by not rushing the TBI individual and his family into seeing the loss "realistically" and by replacing the uncertainty of the future with a focus on understanding the present. These recommendations were implemented in the family support program along with the strategies outlined below.

Reenactment and Expressing Feelings

One of the strategies employed to ameliorate the effects of loss was to provide the TBI clients and their families with a safe venue for expressing intense feelings of anger and guilt. When given the opportunity, the clients and their families expressed a wide variety of emotions (e.g., resentment at the driver of the car that hit them, guilt that they were not wearing motorcycle helmets, anger that they and not their friends were seriously injured). Often these feelings had not been expressed because they conflicted with loyalty to friends and family or were perceived to be socially unacceptable. Acknowledging in therapy that the accident, and its associated losses, was unfair, and that there were no easy answers about why the accident had occurred, often reduced some of the emotional distress. Many of the TBI individuals also found it helpful to revisit the scenes of their injuries around the first anniversary of the accident. Often the activity that led to injury would be repeated (e.g., skiing, motorbike riding, driving to a New Year's party). Some TBI individuals chose to visit places related to the accident (e.g., cemeteries, ski slopes), taking their families with them for support. These "reenactments" occurred spontaneously without any prompting from the therapist.

Graduated Exposure

In a small number of cases, the use of graduated exposure techniques was necessary to prevent the TBI individual from avoiding situations related to some specific aspects of loss (Brasted & Callahan, 1984). Richard's case provides an illustration of the application of this technique.

Graduated Exposure: An Illustrative Case Study

Richard had consistently avoided several social settings (e.g., rugby club, bar, workplace) that were associated with his friend who had died in the accident. He reported that when he had gone to these settings, he had felt as though his friend were standing behind him. Yet when he turned around, there was no one there. These experiences had been frightening and highly aversive. Consequently, he avoided situations in order to prevent any further occurrences of these sensations. An exposure-based intervention was devised in which Richard returned gradually to the situations he had avoided. First, he visited the rugby club, accompanied by a friend. When he could attend the rugby club regularly without anxiety, he returned to his workplace. For the first month, Richard worked in an area that he and his friend had not had contact with. Six weeks later, he returned to his original work area, where he and his friend had been employed prior to the accident. Reassurance and encouragement were provided throughout the process. After approximately 6 months, Richard reported feeling comfortable in these situations, although once every few months he would still feel that his friend was standing behind him.

DEVELOPING A POSITIVE SELF-CONCEPT

The changes in cognitive abilities, personality, and behavior that follow TBI often result in profound changes in self-concept (Tyerman & Humphrey, 1984). Indeed, many of the TBI individuals in the family support program described themselves as being "dumb," "moody," and "selfish" as compared with before the accident. Some TBI individuals felt quite confused about their identity, stating that they no longer knew who they were. These TBI individuals were also frightened that friends and family perceived them as having entirely different personalities as compared to preinjury. Unfortunately, the reestablishment of a positive self-concept was complicated by impaired cognitive skills, which made it difficult for the TBI individuals to self-monitor and analyze their behavior. In order to assist the TBI individuals to re-form a positive self-concept, the methods described below were employed.

The "New You" Concept

The "new you" concept involved helping the TBI individuals form a positive self-image of their postinjury selves. A rationale was provided—namely, that who we are, what we can and cannot do, what we like and do not like, and what our strengths and weaknesses are change over time. At 20, we are not the same as we were at 15, nor are we what we will be at 40. Factors such as age, role changes, and life experiences change us. In the same way, traumatic brain injury also brings change. The challenge is to accept this change and form a new self-image. The TBI clients then engaged in an exercise in which they spent time describing in detail what they were like before the accident (e.g., were they quiet socially or did they enjoy attending loud parties?), what their goals were (e.g., what did they want to do as a career?), what they disliked (e.g., what sort of music did they hate listening to?), what their taste in clothes was, what social activities they enjoyed, and so forth. This information was then compared to their current status. The similarities and differences were elaborated upon, and a list of positive and negative changes was compiled on a worksheet (see Figure 4.4). Listing both positive and negative changes enabled TBI individuals to conceptualize changes in abilities as neutral, rather than purely negative, and helped them appreciate the positive aspects of their "new selves." The worksheet also contained a "No change" column to help TBI individuals identify those aspects of their lives that had remained stable. TBI individuals who perceived that their personalities had totally changed tended to feel quite dissociated, "like I've had a body transplant or am an alien." The recognition of stable patterns of emotions, behavior, and personality from preinjury to postinjury counteracted this dissociative tendency. The aim of this intervention was to establish what Ben-Yishay et al. (1985) refer to as a concept of the "true me."

Improving Self-Appraisal

Chronic negative self-appraisal was a characteristic feature of a subset of the TBI individuals. These individuals consistently saw themselves as stupid, awkward, and foolish, regardless of their actual performance or of the reassurance by

The New Me

Positive changes	Negative changes	No change
More patient	More introverted	Still enjoy cooking and watching videos
Not so selfish	Less social life	Like nature walks
Have spoken at head injury society	More of a perfectionist	Want to have children
Learned how to use a computer	Fatigue	Good at speaking
		Independent

FIGURE 4.4. Sample "new you" worksheet.

others that they had completed a task well. The approach taken to enhance self-appraisal was first to ensure that the TBI individuals were involved in activities at which they were successful. This prevented them from consistently failing at tasks and enabled them to make positive self-appraisals of their performance in at least some of their activities.

After this step, intervention was carried out at a cognitive level. Time was spent helping the TBI individuals form realistic expectations for themselves and reframe their interpretations of their performance. For instance, they were prompted to think about the components of a task that they had completed well (e.g., "I did a good job of cleaning the inside of the car. That's pretty good for the first try since the accident"), rather than make generalized statements about their perceived lack of ability (e.g., "I can't even wash the car right. I'm such an idiot"). They were also encouraged to foster positive self-appraisal by generating positive statements about themselves and repeating these statements to themselves or writing them down for future reference.

Summary of the Procedure for Fostering a Positive Self-Concept

1. Meet with client and present the rationale for the intervention approach (see explanation in text above).
2. Client and therapist discuss in detail the client's preinjury self as reflected in goals, likes and dislikes, personality characteristics, and so forth.
3. Client and therapist discuss in detail the client's postinjury self as reflected in goals, likes and dislikes, personality characteristics, and so forth.
4. Client draws up a list of strengths, paying particular attention to the similarities and differences between pre- and postinjury self. Therapist assists as required.

5. If low self-concept persists, schedule regular successful activities. Monitor these activities.
6. Train client to use cognitive strategies (e.g., cognitive restructuring). Initially provide therapist assistance. This assistance can be faded out over time, as the client learns the strategy.
7. Ask client to generate positive self-statements, assisted by therapist if needed. Self-statements are written down and verbalized, or reviewed by the client on a regular basis.

Developing a Positive Self-Concept: An Illustrative Case Study

Peter, a 29-year-old male, sustained a TBI in a motorcycle accident. His Glasgow Coma Scale score on admission was 11, and he had posttraumatic amnesia lasting 28 days. He sustained diffuse brain injury and a fracture at the base of his skull. After the accident, Peter experienced significant TBI-related sequelae, including mood swings, depression, chronic fatigue, and slowness of information processing. These impairments delayed his return to work and his ability to relate to others. He also displayed problems with negative self-concept that were exacerbating his depression. The focus of his concern was his body image, which he perceived to have changed after the accident. He felt that his stomach, his nose, and his buttocks protruded. In social situations, he was conscious of this perception and would frequently blush, which caused him further distress. Figure 4.5 is a picture he sketched in response to the prompt "Draw what you look like." The nose, the stomach, and the blushing are all prominent features. In order to cope with his negative body image, he had begun to exercise daily to lose weight. This practice, however, caused increased tiredness and resulted in further vulnerability to low mood. His weight had not in fact changed since he had been discharged from the hospital and was actually less than it had been before the accident.

Discussion with Peter about his beliefs revealed that for him, physical attractiveness was closely associated with success in the workplace, approval of others, and the ability to have a positive relationship with a woman. He felt that he had lost the ability to reach any of these goals because of the TBI, and thus he embarked on a program of increasing his attractiveness in an attempt to regain at least part of his lost potential. The association between attractiveness and success was challenged, and Peter was given an assignment to identify examples of unattractive successful people and unsuccessful attractive people over the next week. Peter was also helped to identify his strengths and the positive aspects of his personality by discussing them with the therapist and writing them down. Within 3 weeks, Peter had decreased his amount of exercise and no longer felt that his body was distorted.

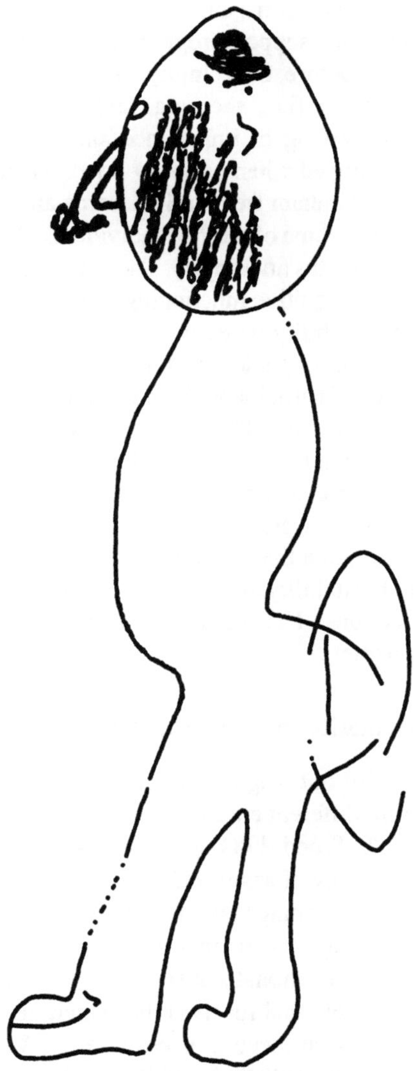

FIGURE 4.5. Drawing of physical self-concept.

MANAGEMENT OF ANGER AND IRRITABILITY

Irritability and anger problems are commonly reported following traumatic brain injury (e.g., Hinkeldey & Corrigan, 1990; McKinlay et al., 1981). Certainly, all the TBI clients in the family support program reported increased irritability and anger as compared with before their injury. This irritability did not always manifest itself as overt anger (i.e., shouting, feelings of rage), but was rather described as a persistent feeling of impatience and becoming annoyed easily. Annette became easily annoyed when her baby cried, Richard was irritable with his mother and sister, and Graham frequently became angry with his workmates when they spoke loudly. For some of the TBI individuals, the anger and irritability decreased in the first few months after injury. These early improvements appeared to be related to recovery of cognitive functioning. Richard, for instance, displayed significant decreases in irritability when he became able to track the content of conversations and could better understand what was happening around him. Nevertheless, the majority of participants found that anger and irritability continued even up to 2 years postinjury. The most common precipitant of anger and irritability appeared to be interactions with other people (e.g., being told by a partner that you are not able to drive), environmental noises (e.g., sound of children playing, television), physical discomfort (e.g., feeling too hot, stubbing a toe), and slow service (e.g., in a line at the bank). The following sections discuss the etiology of anger and irritability and describe the intervention techniques used to ameliorate these emotions. The modification of aggressive behavior is discussed separately in Chapter 5.

Mediation of Anger and Irritability

As many authors point out, anger and irritability are not unitary emotions; rather, they can arise from different etiologies, both neurological and psychological (Haffey & Scibak, 1989; Wood, 1984) (see Table 4.1). The neurological factors commonly cited in the etiology of anger and irritability include the posttraumatic epilepsy and the frontal lobe damage (Wood, 1987). The psychological explanations for anger encompass anger as an emotional reaction to the losses that occur following TBI (e.g., loss of vocational status), anger as a learned behavior that is reinforced when the TBI individual receives its desired outcome, and anger as a goal-directed behavior aimed at meeting needs (Haffey & Scibak, 1989; Wood, 1987). According to Prigatano (1992), irritability and anger are not necessarily related to neurological impairment, but may in some cases constitute a reactionary behavioral disturbance. This assertion is based on research indicating that irritability correlates significantly with forgetfulness, being tired when other people are around, and having difficulty following conversations (Hinkeldey & Corrigan, 1990).

TABLE 4.1. Expression of Anger and Irritability

Psychological mediation	Neurological mediation	
Goal-directed behavior	Epileptogenic behavior	Frontal aggression
Provoked and goal-directed	Unprovoked	Provoked and directed toward source of provocation
Aware of actions when angry	Not always aware of actions when angry	Aware of actions when angry
Some control once angry	Little or no control once angry	Little or no control once angry

Implementing Preventative Strategies

As it was usually possible to identify antecedent "triggers" for irritability and anger, preventative measures could be put in place. The simplest preventative strategy was to advise participants to avoid situations that were associated with a high risk of irritability or anger occurring. Annette, for instance, often became angry with her sister when she arrived home tired from going shopping. Hence, she was advised to avoid her sister when either of them was fatigued. Other preventative strategies included taking regular prescheduled rest breaks, taking deep breaths before entering trigger situations, and making modifications to routines or environments. Hamish had repeatedly been irritable with his children at breakfast time. This had caused considerable tension within the family. Simply asking his wife to be responsible for breakfast time and asking Hamish to help the children at dinnertime markedly reduced Hamish's irritability in the mornings. Similarly, ensuring that Simon was not exposed to multiple stimuli (e.g., television sounds, children, lights) when he arrived home reduced his irritability. In some instances, it was necessary to provide the TBI individual with practical assistance. Susan, for example, was becoming increasingly irritable with her baby son when he cried. A nurse came to help her on a part-time basis for several months. When Susan's ability to cope with the baby's crying improved, the nurse's hours were gradually decreased until this assistance was completely withdrawn.

Modifying expectations also proved to be an important preventative strategy. As DeBoskey and Morin (1985) point out, anger and irritability can arise when TBI individuals discover that they are unable to perform simple tasks effectively. The experience of failure often leads to intense frustration. In such situations, it was necessary to help the TBI individuals readjust their expectations so that they were able to perceive their performance as successful. For example, Graham's irritability at work arose from his unrealistically high expectations about the amount of work he should be able to do in a day. When he failed to meet these expectations, he became irritable. Lowering his expectations about the amount of work he could complete was associated with a reduction in Graham's level of irritability.

Summary of the Procedure for Reducing Anger and Irritability

1. Avoid high-risk situations in which feelings of anger and irritability are likely to be experienced (e.g., discussing financial problems with a family member who is very tired).
2. Take prescheduled rest breaks (e.g., 10 minutes' rest every hour).
3. Modify routines (e.g., if irritable later in the evening, schedule children's bath time for before the evening meal).
4. Modify the environment (e.g., reduce the presence of multiple stimuli by turning off lights, television, or radio).
5. Provide practical assistance (e.g., home help, gardening, financial aid).
6. Assist the TBI client to readjust his expectations so that he does not always "fail" and become frustrated.

Skills Training

When goals are not met, people incline toward one of two responses. The first response is to select an alternative approach in order to achieve the goal. The alternative response is to become angry and frustrated or to try to avoid the situation (Haffey & Scibak, 1989). One of the primary aims of the skills-training intervention was to teach a range of coping strategies that could be used when participants were unable to meet their goals. Families and TBI individuals were taught to use problem-solving strategies to utilize the simple relaxation techniques described earlier in this chapter, to communicate to others about how they were feeling, and, where appropriate, to take time out if they were becoming angry (e.g., Annette left the situation and watched television for 10 minutes). When anger and irritability were a serious problem, a stress-inoculation approach based upon the Lira et al. (1983) model was employed. This approach involves three phases: (1) *cognitive preparation*, in which the participants were provided with education about anger, taught how to recognize angry feelings, and instructed how to identify high-risk situations; (2) *skills acquisition*, in which participants learned skills such as the ability to reevaluate anger-provoking situations, relaxation, and time out; (3) *application training*, in which the participants developed a hierarchy of anger-provoking situations. The situations were role played with the therapist, and the participants practiced the skills that had been taught. When the participants were proficient in dealing with the situations in a role-play context, they then proceeded to practice the skills in everyday life.

To assist TBI individuals to recall coping strategies, the McKinlay and Hickox (1988) ANGER protocol was taught: Anticipate the trigger situations,

Notice the signs of rising anger, Go and use coping strategies (e.g., relaxation techniques, self-statements), Extract yourself from the situation, Record how you coped. Note down the lessons learned for next time. Some participants wrote this protocol on a cue card that they carried in their pockets and referred to during the day.

Advice to Families

Families were quite understandably concerned when the TBI individual became angry or irritable. Some families described feeling as though they were "walking on eggshells," constantly striving to anticipate the factors that would cause the TBI sufferer to be angry, in the hope that they might modify the situation and hence avert the anger. However, determining what it is that frustrates a TBI individual is often difficult because the cognitive, perceptual, and memory difficulties that lead to the frustration are often underestimated by families and health professionals alike (Prigatano, 1992). Other families became intensely frustrated themselves, particularly with the low-level irritability of the TBI individuals, which in many instances persisted for weeks and was manifested as a short temper, oppositional behavior, and sarcastic comments. Families were informed that irritability is a common TBI-related sequela, given reassurance that their own feelings of frustration with the TBI individual were very normal, and provided with the advice outlined below.

Summary of Advice to Families

1. When possible, always allow the individual to make choices and be involved in decision making. Doing so reduces the likelihood that irritability and anger will occur.
2. Do not directly confront the TBI individual when he is angry. Try to distract him with another activity, leave him alone if possible, or gently ask him to take some "time out."
3. When practical, ignore verbal outbursts. Use this as a signal to implement a preventative strategy.
4. Try not to fight back by yelling or hitting. Doing so only makes the situation worse.
5. When the situation has calmed down, communicate clearly with the TBI individual about what went wrong, how it made you feel, and what you would like to change (e.g., "Mark, remember that argument over whether you could buy those shoes? Well, I felt quite embarrassed by your language. Next time, can you let me know how you feel without swearing? I'd really appreciate that").
6. At all times, protect yourself and your children. Leave the situation if it is

dangerous. Have a backup person who is prepared to come in and help you should things get out of hand.

7. Maintain contact with some friends (or a counselor) with whom you can let off steam and express how you feel.

MANAGING CATASTROPHIC REACTIONS

The concept of catastrophic reactions following brain injury was first introduced by Kurt Goldstein (1952). A catastrophic reaction can be loosely defined as an extreme emotional response to relatively mild stressors. For example, as soon as Keith found that his insurance payment was less than expected, he became severely depressed. When spoken to on the telephone an hour after receiving the notification letter, he stated, "I should have finished it off. I might as well have died in the car." Later that day, when he discovered he had misread the letter, his mood returned to normal. Similarly, when Graham found out that he was not able to complete the plumbing he was working on, he became suicidal and was seen carrying two guns by his sister, who then rushed him to his doctor. Three days later, his mood was stable and he was embarrassed by his actions. Other participants had similarly extreme reactions to a diverse range of situations such as changes in living situations, receiving bad haircuts, and being served poorly cooked meals.

Characteristically, the TBI individual became extremely anxious or depressed, rational decision making was impaired, and a number of health professionals, friends, and family members became involved as the individual contacted them for help. Catastrophic reactions occurred in only a subset of the participants. These individuals tended to be characterized by depressive symptomatology, poor impulse control associated with frontal lobe damage, and more severe injuries (i.e., posttraumatic amnesia longer than 10 days). The speed with which the catastrophic change occurred was often remarkable in that a seemingly stable person would become severely emotionally distressed within hours. Mood would then return to normal within a few days if the triggering problem was successfully resolved.

Intervention for catastrophic reactions first involved ensuring the safety of the TBI individual, especially if there was a risk of suicide. Usually, the individual went to stay with family or friends, although one individual had to be admitted to the hospital. After safety had been ensured, the initial triggering problem was resolved. For instance, if the catastrophic reaction had been triggered by a disagreement with a workmate, the TBI individual was prompted to speak to the person and resolve the issue as soon as possible. Experience demonstrated that this procedure was more effective than focusing on the emotional distress itself, as the distress dissipated quickly once the original problem was dealt with. Initial assistance was quite directive, with the therapist providing clear guidelines regarding the decisions that were required (e.g., if the individual needed to go to stay with a friend, or if he needed to contact his employer and request sick leave).

Support and encouragement were provided to the family, who were naturally enough often very concerned. Liaison with the other health professionals also proved vital in ensuring that a consistent approach to the management of the catastrophic reaction was adopted. When handled in this way, the TBI individual's mood would often rapidly return to normal and he would be ready to resume his daily activities within a week. After the catastrophic reaction was resolved, time was spent with the TBI individual and his family discussing what had happened and formulating a preventative plan for dealing with similar situations in the future. In most cases, catastrophic reactions occurred repeatedly. However, when the TBI individual and family learned more adaptive ways of coping with catastrophic reactions, the reactions became less frequent and less severe.

Summary of the Procedure for Managing Catastrophic Reactions

1. Ensure that the TBI individual is physically safe.
2. Take steps to help the TBI individual resolve the crisis that triggered the catastrophic reaction. The use of problem-solving procedures is helpful in determining the steps that need to be taken in order to resolve the crisis.
3. Provide advice if any important decisions need to be made (e.g., if the TBI individual is deciding whether to leave his job).
4. Contact family and offer support and reassurance.
5. Liaise with all other health professionals involved.

FOSTERING AWARENESS

One of the most demanding problems faced by health professionals involved in the management of TBI patients is dealing with the patients' lack of awareness regarding neuropsychological impairment (Youngjohn & Altman, 1989). Some authors see this lack of awareness as a direct result of organically based cognitive impairment (e.g., Ben-Yishay et al., 1985; Gobble et al., 1987), while others see it as a resistant behavioral syndrome (e.g., Youngjohn & Altman, 1989) or as an emotional response designed to avoid the anxiety and grief that accompany awareness of deficit (e.g., Deaton, 1986; Ridley, 1989). Recent findings have shown that TBI individuals' degree of insight does improve over time (Godfrey et al., 1993b), that their level of denial is not related to severity of cognitive deficit (McKinlay & Brooks, 1984), and that significantly higher levels of depression are found in those who are aware of their neuropsychological impairments (Boake et al., 1987). For these reasons, the family support program conceptualized lack of awareness as an emotional coping response (see also Moore et al., 1989). However, the possibility of organically mediated anosognosia was carefully considered on a case-by-case basis.

The rationale for attempting to improve awareness was that a realistic appreciation of neuropsychological impairment would lead to improved motivation for rehabilitation, greater implementation of compensatory strategies, and improved ability to set realistic goals (McGlynn, 1990). Certainly, it appeared that failure to recognize and accept neuropsychological impairment led to considerable emotional distress and delayed the process of readjustment. Patrick, for example, was unable to accept that he could no longer run his own painting business. This lack of acceptance led to months of heartbreaking attempts at work resulting in failure. The challenge was, as Ben-Yishay et al. (1985, p. 255) put it, "to become aware of one's problems, without being overwhelmed by this knowledge, and without having one's morale and determination to work hard to overcome them shattered." Interventions for improving awareness are designed to be utilized in a graduated manner. The initial intervention approaches were less intrusive and confrontational. Only when these approaches failed were direct feedback and planned self-discovery used. As Ylvisaker and Szekeres (1989) point out, direct feedback techniques are indicated only if the TBI individual or family members are not benefitting from experience and months or years after injury show a lack of awareness of impairment. At all times, the therapist carefully monitored the participant's emotional status to ensure that the potential threat to self-worth from intervention did not precipitate depression (Youngjohn & Altman, 1989). This four-step intervention procedure is referred to as *guided realization* and is described below.

Level 1: Providing Information

Presenting information to TBI patients and their families about TBI sequelae is a common method of assisting them to form realistic expectations and attitudes (e.g., Fordyce & Roueche, 1986; Klonoff & Prigatano, 1987). All participants in the family support program received comprehensive education that described the nature of their injury and the possible long-term effects. The education procedure is described in detail in Chapter 6. Education was used to illustrate, in a nonthreatening manner, potential performance difficulties that the TBI individual might experience (see also Gobble et al., 1987). In most cases, the practical consequences of neuropsychological impairment were illustrated (e.g., memory deficits can result in difficulty completing tasks at work). Neuropsychological symptoms were normalized using examples from "other people who have had traumatic brain injuries." This educational strategy created a distance between the individual's own personal situation and the example that was being given. The aim of creating this distance was to allow the TBI individual to consider the potential impact of neuropsychological impairment without having to acknowledge that he himself was experiencing these difficulties. Education also served to promote discussion between TBI individuals and their family members regarding the nature of their neuropsychological symptoms.

Level 2: Hierarchical Questioning

In recognition that questioning techniques can enhance the process of self-appraisal (Cicerone, 1989), hierarchical questioning was also employed to improve TBI individuals' awareness. Hierarchical questioning involved asking increasingly specific questions to help TBI individuals and their families identify changes that had occurred as a result of the TBI individuals' injuries. Initial questions were very general two-step inquiries such as "How was your memory before the accident?" and "What is it like now?" If the participant remained unaware of any deficits when this questioning approach was used, a more specific question that included an example was asked—for instance: "Do you forget what people have said to you?" When this approach repeatedly failed to elicit any awareness of impairment, the TBI individual was asked to describe an incident that clearly demonstrated his difficulties (e.g., "Tell me about last week when you forgot what the time of our appointment was"). Asking the individual to answer the questions from other points of view also proved to be a very effective strategy (e.g., "Do you think that your wife would say that you had a memory problem? What makes you think she would say that?").

Summary of the Procedure for Hierarchical Questioning

Step 1. Ask a general question.
Example: Use very general two-step inquiries such as "How was your memory before the accident?" and "What is it like now?"

Step 2. Ask a specific question.
Example: Ask a more specific question that includes an example—for instance: "Do you forget what people have said to you?"

Step 3. Describe an incident.
Example: When the specific questioning approach fails to elicit any awareness of impairment, ask the TBI individual to describe an incident that will clearly demonstrate his difficulty.

Step 4. Explain other people's points of view.
Example: Ask the TBI individual to ask questions from other people's points of view (e.g., "Do you think that your wife would say that you had a memory problem? What makes you think she would say that?").

All questioning was carried out in a neutral manner during routine family support sessions. Below are listed examples of hierarchal questioning as applied to five different problems. The incidents listed are based upon real-life examples that arose during the family support sessions. The purpose of hierarchical questioning was to encourage TBI individuals to develop awareness without having to directly confront them regarding their neuropsychological impairments.

Examples of Hierarchical Questioning

Socialization

General question: What's your social life like these days?
Specific question: When did you last go out to see friends?
Incident: I thought you'd refused to go out and see friends . . . ?

Marital relationship

General question: How are things going between you and your wife?
Specific question: Some people find they are more interested in sex after a brain injury. Has this happened to you?
Incident: You told me that your partner is not very enthusiastic in bed?

Judgment

General question: Have you done things without thinking?
Specific question: What happened with the dog?
Incident: Didn't an advertisement for the dog appear in the paper and your wife didn't know about it?

Parenting

General question: How are things going with the kids?
Specific question: Do you think you get quite impatient with [child's name]?
Incident: Umm . . . I thought I saw you yelling at [child's name] because she wanted to go to the toilet?

Motivation

General question: What do you do with your free time?
Specific question: Are you doing anything to help at home?
Incident: I got the impression that the television was on for most of the day?

Level 3: Feedback

The use of feedback to promote insight and awareness has received considerable attention in the literature (e.g., Fordyce & Roueche, 1986; Klonoff et al., 1989; Ylvisaker & Szekeres, 1989). The usual feedback protocol involves asking the TBI individual to complete a task (e.g., taking a memory test or having a brief conversation with a stranger) and then providing feedback on his performance. Sometimes the TBI individual is shown a video of his performance, and his performance shortcomings are pointed out. Feedback can also be delivered by computers, family members, health professionals, and in the context of group therapy (Deaton, 1986). There is some empirical evidence that the provision of feedback decreases inappropriate sexual behavior (Burke et al., 1991), increases the consistency between staff and patient ratings of performance (Fordyce & Roueche, 1986), and improves TBI individuals' ability to estimate their performance on cognitive tasks (Youngjohn & Altman, 1989). However, feedback is best given in the context of a supportive ongoing relationship with the therapist and in a neutral manner (Klonoff et al., 1989). In the family support program, direct verbal feedback about the TBI individuals' deficits was provided only when the informational approach and hierarchical questioning had proven ineffective.

The most frequently used feedback technique involved reinforcing insightful comments made by the TBI individuals. Aaron, for example, had become verbose and verbally disinhibited after his injury. On one occasion, he correctly commented, "I'm talking silly, aren't I?" He was immediately praised by the therapist for his awareness, and means of improving the conversation were then discussed. For a minority of participants, it was necessary to give direct feedback about their performance (e.g., "It seems that your reaction time is slow when you ride the motorbike"). The most common source of direct feedback was family members, and their feedback proved extremely effective. Derek began doing regular household chores after his brother candidly told him that he was not completing the tasks that he was assigned. Up until that time, Derek had been unaware that any problem existed. Clinical experience has suggested that feedback is a positive technique. However, it needs to be delivered by someone whom the TBI individual can communicate with well, concrete examples of the problem must be provided, and feedback needs to be interspersed with a focus on the positive aspects of the individual's achievements.

Every opportunity was taken to encourage the higher-functioning participants to evaluate their own performance, taking into consideration TBI-related deficits. Peter, for instance, was advised to provide himself with feedback regarding his work performance and its relationship to his mood disturbance. Therapist coaching was required initially, but was gradually faded out over time.

Level 4: Planned Self-Discovery

The planned self-discovery technique was based upon the Ylvisaker and Szekeres (1989) "directed self-discovery" method, in which TBI individuals plan a series of tasks and brainstorm with the therapist to identify possible factors that might prevent and facilitate goal accomplishment. This technique was extended to incorporate the provision of feedback on a series of tasks that had been set for the TBI individuals to test their assumptions regarding their level of skill. For example, early after his discharge from the hospital, Joseph became easily disoriented in town. His parents were concerned that he would get lost when he went out. However, Joseph maintained that his sense of direction was excellent and was frustrated and angry at his parents' desire to accompany him when he left the house. Joseph did not accept feedback about his difficulties with poor sense of direction from either the psychologist or his occupational therapist. Therefore, a task was devised whereby Joseph was left in the city for 30 minutes, after which his mother met him at a prearranged place. This demonstrated to Joseph that he did indeed have difficulty with his sense of direction. Similar tasks of increasing difficulty continued to be used intermittently as "practice" (e.g., being left in a different place from that where he was picked up). The use of these practice tasks facilitated assessment of his performance level. When he was able to complete the more complicated tasks successfully, he was then allowed to go out independently without his parents becoming concerned.

Summary of the Procedure for Planned Self-Discovery

Step 1. Determine the area to be targeted.
Example: Paul is adamant that he is able to work full time as an engineer, although his vocational guidance officer has determined that he is not work-ready.

Step 2. Set a task to test the TBI individual's assumptions about his performance.
Example: Set up a work trial for Paul.

Step 3. Ensure that the situation is safe.
Example: Arrange the work trial for one day only. Arrange for supervision to be available.

Step 4. Ensure that the TBI individual is given a task that demonstrates his impairment, but that is not so totally beyond his capacity that he risks becoming depressed.
Example: Arrange for Paul to work assembling machinery rather than designing machinery.

Step 5. Inform the family about the purpose and procedure of planned discovery.
Example: Visit Paul's family and discuss the work trial.

Step 6. Present the task as an "experiment" and predict failure. This ensures that the TBI individual can experience failure without loss of self-respect.
Example: Tell Paul that he is not actually expected to be able to complete a day's work, but that rather than arguing about the issue, an experiment has been set up.

Step 7. Ask the TBI individual to write down what he expects his level of performance to be.
Example: Ask Paul to estimate how long he thinks he can work and what he thinks the quality and pace of his work will be.

Step 8. Ask the TBI individual to compare his actual performance to his estimated performance.
Example: Ask Paul to compare his estimated hours worked vs. actual hours worked.

Step 9. Ask other significant individuals to provide feedback.
Example: Assist Paul's supervisor to give feedback. Ask Paul's family about his behavior and fatigue level when he returned from work.

Step 10. Reinforce any improvement in awareness.
Example: Tell Paul that you are impressed that he has recognized that he does get tired easily.

Step 11. Acknowledge that performance does improve over time and arrange for a review.
Example: A review set for 3 months later on the recommendation of the vocational guidance officer.

IMPLEMENTING INTERVENTIONS TO ENHANCE EMOTIONAL ADJUSTMENT

The implementation of interventions to enhance emotional adjustment required considerable time and therapeutic creativity. Some TBI individuals did not have any conceptual framework for labeling emotions or for constructively expressing feelings. This lack meant that they needed to be taught how to identify emotions before any further intervention could be carried out. It was found to be critical to use concrete examples and utilize metaphors that were meaningful to the TBI individuals and their families. For instance, the family of one participant had a saying that their family were like "weeds," in that weeds are strong and will always grow back. This metaphor proved to be highly effective for the TBI client when he wanted to motivate himself during episodes of depression.

Other useful strategies to increase understanding of emotional concepts included using drawings to overcome language problems (Prigatano et al., 1986b), being relatively structured and directive when implementing interventions (Cicerone, 1989; Gobble et al., 1987), and presenting information repeatedly (Rosenthal, 1989). The use of cognitive strategies appeared to be most effective with the highly functioning participants, while the behavioral techniques proved to be more useful for those TBI individuals with global cognitive impairment and families who had little previous experience in identifying and modifying emotions.

5

Improving Social Competency

Traumatic brain injury (TBI) is frequently associated with impaired social competency. TBI individuals may become too talkative, make socially inappropriate comments, speak too loudly, or fail to adequately consider other people's feelings and wishes. Characteristics such as these can have a profound impact on all aspects of the TBI individual's social role functioning (e.g., vocational adjustment, marital satisfaction, peer relationships). Indeed, there is hardly any aspect of life that is not affected as a result of impaired social competency (Helffenstein & Wechsler, 1982). In acknowledgment of the critical role that social competency plays in adjustment following TBI, the family support program included interventions designed to enhance social competency. This chapter describes these intervention strategies.

INTERPERSONAL-SKILLS TRAINING

Deficits in interpersonal skills have been observed in a large proportion of individuals with brain injuries (Spence et al., 1993). Both verbal and nonverbal communication skills (e.g., appropriate use of eye contact, ability to take turns) may be impaired (Brotherton et al., 1988; Giles et al., 1988), as may be social cognition (Lezak, 1978). Interpersonal-skills deficits may reflect preinjury level of social skills, emotional factors such as the fear of negative evaluation, and cognitive impairment such as the lack of a set of cognitive guidelines to shape and direct social behavior (Brotherton et al., 1988; Helffenstein & Wechsler, 1982; Malkmus, 1989). A wide range of skills deficits were evident in TBI participants in the family support program, including overtalkativeness, inappropriate conversational content (e.g., constant focus on self, providing sexually explicit information), and impaired expression (e.g., lack of sufficient variation in tonal modulation, excessively loud vocalization).

Intervention to ameliorate interpersonal-skills deficits began with an observational assessment. TBI individuals were observed by the therapist as they participated in a conversation with family members, with a friend, or with a health professional. During this interaction, the therapist rated the TBI individual's interaction skill level. The Profile of Functional Impairment in Communication (Linscott, Knight, & Godfrey, 1993) provides a comprehensive scale for assessing interpersonal competency following TBI and is presented in Appendix B. Following the assessment, a list of target behaviors was compiled. Peter, for example, had been told by his brother that he talked too much and was boring people. These problems had also been observed by the therapist. Hence, the quantity of his speech and the egocentric nature of its content were targeted for intervention. Once a target behavior had been identified, the therapist gave feedback to the TBI individual about the behavior and explained why it needed to be modified. Alternative behaviors were taught and modeled, and the TBI individual then engaged in a series of role plays with the therapist during which the new skills were practiced and feedback on the TBI individual's performance was given.

Peter, for instance, was taught how to monitor another person's level of interest in the content of his conversation (e.g., by checking whether the person is fidgeting, not making eye contact, or not asking questions), role plays were carried out in which he was asked to identify "boredom signals," and modeling was employed to demonstrate how to increase the other person's involvement in a conversation (e.g., by asking open questions). These skills were then practiced in a role play, and specific feedback was provided on his performance (e.g., the degree to which he was talking too much). He was also taught how to discriminate social situations in which it was appropriate to disclose personal information (e.g., details about his accident and its consequences). This process of assessment, feedback, skills acquisition, modeling, and skill rehearsal has been employed by several other workers in the field of TBI rehabilitation and has been empirically validated as an effective means of enhancing interpersonal skills (e.g., Helffenstein & Wechsler, 1982; Brotherton et al., 1988).

Another helpful technique designed to improve interpersonal skills was self-monitoring. Schloss et al. (1985) provide an excellent example of this technique. In their study, they provided three TBI individuals with a mechanical counter to record the number of questions they asked during a conversation with another person. The TBI individuals also monitored the number of compliments they paid the other person and the number of statements concerning themselves they made to the other person. The effect of the self-monitoring was to increase the number of compliments the TBI individuals paid the other person and to decrease the level of self-disclosure. This process was used in a modified form as part of the family support program and was found to be very useful. Joseph, for instance, had trouble controlling his laughter. He had been informed by his younger sister that he laughed too much and was laughing at things that were not funny. In order to better self-monitor his laughter, he was taught to use his watch to check that he was not laughing for more than 10 seconds at a time. As a result, the frequency and duration of his inappropriate laughing rapidly declined.

INCREASING SOCIAL CONTACT

According to Thomsen (1984), the greatest subjective burden for TBI individuals following injury is their lack of social contact. The decline in social contact following TBI appears to be related to the TBI patient's inability to maintain preinjury behavior patterns and roles (Wagner et al., 1990). Friends will tolerate behavioral problems (e.g., irritability and mood swings) for several months, but eventually tend to distance themselves from the TBI individual. Hence, TBI individuals often lose preinjury friends and subsequently have great difficulty in developing new close friendships (Kinsella, Ford, & Moran, 1989). The need for social contact may consequently be directed toward family members who begin to form the primary support network for the TBI individual. This role can prove burdensome for families who are required to provide continuing emotional support for the TBI individual (Kinsella et al., 1989). The TBI individual's level of satisfaction with his social network is important as a mediator of his perceived level of functioning and recovery following TBI (Wagner et al., 1990).

In the family support program, significant decreases in the TBI individual's level of social contact and number of friends occurred in approximately one third of the group. The reasons for these decreases were diverse, and included social-skills deficits, anxiety, poor self-esteem, low levels of motivation, and adverse personality changes. Joseph, for example, avoided his classmates because he was unsure whether he would be able to maintain a conversation with them. Peter decreased his level of social contact because of his anxiety about his inability to remember even close friends' names. Derek avoided women because he perceived he was no longer attractive, and Keith stayed at home because he could no longer drink with his friends.

Both behavioral and cognitive strategies were used to extend the TBI individuals' social networks. From the first point of contact, the importance of maintaining previous relationships and establishing new ones was emphasized. Friends were encouraged to visit the TBI individual, and they were given information regarding traumatic brain injury. Participants were also questioned about their level of social contact at each follow-up visit. If it was found that the TBI individuals' social contact levels had reduced, they were encouraged to set a goal to spend more time with friends.

When the TBI individual had serious difficulties in maintaining an adequate social network, more structured interventions were put in place. These usually involved setting a goal for social contact (e.g., going to the movies with a friend).

These goals were set on a weekly or biweekly basis and were monitored regularly. Any difficulties in achieving the goals were discussed, and any necessary changes were implemented. Joseph, for example, had difficulty finding sufficient opportunity to practice conversation skills. Assessment indicated that he had actually been avoiding situations involving social contact. After this problem was discussed with him, it was agreed that he would remain with his classmates for lunch instead of returning home. Doing so provided him with increased opportunity for social contact and, as well, increased his opportunity to practice conversation skills.

In many cases, goal setting needed to be supplemented with the use of cognitive restructuring strategies. Participants often felt that others no longer liked them or that they were no longer socially acceptable. These beliefs needed to be challenged before TBI individuals would engage in greater social contact. Richard, for example, felt that his friends no longer enjoyed his company, even though they continued to phone him and ask him to participate in activities with them. He simply attributed this to their "pitying" him and therefore refused to go. After he examined this belief in more detail, he recognized that it was actually untrue. This change in thinking paved the way for greater social contact with his friends. Developing new friendships also required that some participants change their maladaptive social cognitions. For instance, after his accident, Keith no longer wanted to spend time with his old friends, who were heavily involved with alcohol and drugs. However, he was unable to conceive that he could make friends with persons with any other interests. Considerable time was spent discussing his choice of friends with him. With ongoing therapist encouragement, he discovered that he could relate to some of the younger married men in the community, and he proceeded to establish a friendship with one of them.

Summary of the Procedure for Increasing Social Contact

1. From the time of the first meeting with the client and the family, reinforce the importance of social contact.
2. Encourage the client's friends to visit the client in the hospital. Provide the friends with education regarding TBI, offer support, and answer any questions they may have.
3. After the client's discharge from the hospital, monitor whether the client has regular social contact. The monitoring needs to occur at every visit, and involves obtaining specific information about the client's social activity during the period since the last visit (e.g., number of visitors, number of social activities engaged in outside the home).
4. On each visit, prompt the client to maintain social contacts. Discuss any plans the client has made for social contact before the next visit.
5. Compliment the client when he has maintained social contacts.

6. If the client has difficulties with decreasing social contact, decreasing leisure activities, or decreasing numbers of friends, carry out a careful assessment to determine the cause of the problem (e.g., low motivation, social-skills deficits).
7. Implement intervention strategies on the basis of the assessment. Common interventions include goal setting and interpersonal-skills training.
8. Where necessary, utilize cognitive intervention strategies. First, assist the client to identify the cognitions that are preventing him from engaging in social contact (e.g., "I'm boring and no one likes being with a boring person"). Second, use questioning techniques to challenge these beliefs and cognitions (e.g., "How do you know that no one likes you?"). Third, aid the client to develop more appropriate cognitions (e.g., "I'm doing okay. My friends have asked me to go out with them, so they must want my company"). This is a long process. The therapist may need to assist in generating replacement statements. Writing the statements down, and both rehearsing them aloud and having the client rehearse them mentally, can aid effective implementation.

ENCOURAGING INVOLVEMENT IN LEISURE PURSUITS

The number of leisure and recreational pursuits an individual is able to participate in is often decreased as a consequence of TBI (Thomsen, 1984). TBI individuals in the family support program were forced to stop participating in a wide variety of their preinjury leisure activities because of medical complications, reduced skill due to TBI-related impairment, or the risk of incurring a second injury. Examples of lost recreational activities included horse riding, motorcycle riding, judo, scuba diving, rugby, basketball, and ballroom dancing. When these important leisure pursuits were discontinued, the TBI individuals' levels of social contact with friends drastically diminished, as did their general satisfaction with their social life. Hence, it proved important to assist the TBI individuals to involve themselves in alternative leisure pursuits.

The first step toward increasing the TBI individuals' participation in leisure pursuits was to help them generate a list of potential enjoyable leisure activities. Generating such lists proved to be particularly problematic in small rural towns, where the majority of leisure activities revolved around the consumption of alcohol. The TBI individuals had been advised against alcohol consumption; surprisingly, all but two participants complied with this advice. The two TBI individuals who drank alcohol reduced their consumption substantially compared with before their injury. As a result of their decision not to consume alcohol, many of the TBI individuals felt uncomfortable in social settings, especially when their friends got drunk while they remained sober. This social discomfort resulted in avoidance of alcohol-related activities. Despite this emphasis on alcohol, it was possible to plan some alcohol-free leisure activities involving physical exercise. Physical sports such as swimming, golf, yachting, attending a gym, and playing badminton all proved to be successful alternatives to activities involving consumption of alcohol. Important to the process of increasing involvement in leisure pursuits was the discovery of new activities that were similar to those engaged in before the accident. Richard, for example, was unable to ride his motorcycle; however, he became an avid spectator at races and read many motorcycle magazines. Similarly, Grant, though unable to play rugby, was able to become the rugby team manager.

Once potential leisure activities had been determined, goals were set. Goals were monitored regularly, and the number of leisure activities the TBI individual engaged in was gradually increased across time. Having a close friend or relative accompany the TBI individual proved helpful, as it increased the likelihood that the TBI individual would engage in the activity.

Summary of the Procedure for Increasing Involvement in Leisure Pursuits

1. The TBI individual and the therapist generate a list of potential leisure activities.
2. Goals are set for the level of participation in the leisure activities.
3. Family and friends are encouraged to accompany the TBI individual in the leisure activities. Over time, family involvement is faded out so that the TBI individual eventually independently organizes and engages in appropriate leisure pursuits.
4. Progress is monitored. The TBI individual is complimented when goals are met.

Figure 5.1 displays single-case outcome data for an intervention aimed at increasing the number of social activities that Graham participated in. Baseline recording demonstrated that in the weeks prior to intervention, he was engaging in no social activities whatsoever. Assessment indicated that there was a temporal association between his mood, his number of work hours, and his level of social activity. In those weeks during which he worked long hours and engaged in no social activity, he became severely depressed. Reducing work hours and increasing leisure activities resulted in markedly improved mood. It was decided, on the basis of this temporal association, to increase his number of leisure activities. Engaging in leisure activities had the advantage that recreation was incompatible with working excessive hours. Graham and his sister generated a list of activities (e.g., yachting, going fishing). Initially, Graham's leisure goal was to participate in one activity per week; however, this goal was soon achieved, and Graham set a

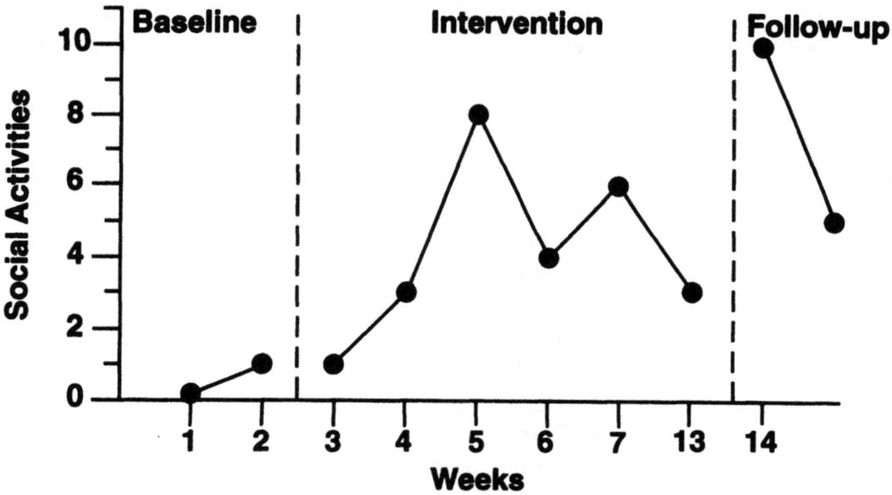

FIGURE 5.1. Frequency of social activities.

new goal of four activities each week. Graham exceeded even this target, and gains were maintained at 6 and 7 weeks follow-up. Goal setting was reinstated several months later, when Graham again increased his work hours and reduced his leisure activities.

ASSISTING VOCATIONAL ADJUSTMENT

In the United States, up to two thirds of individuals who have sustained a severe TBI are unlikely to be competitively employed (Wehman et al., 1989a). The cost of the failure to return to competitive employment is high, both financially in terms of lost income and emotionally in terms of reduced self-esteem (Kreutzer et al., 1991). Reduced vocational status also forces role changes to occur within families as TBI individuals spend more time within the home and partners are obliged to join the work force or extend their working hours.

The barriers that prevent TBI individuals' returning to their occupations are many. Slowness of information processing, lack of punctuality, disinhibited behavior, memory impairment, poor initiation skills, physical disability, behavioral problems, transportation difficulties, inability to plan tasks, and insufficient interpersonal skill all impact upon the TBI individual's employability. While employers may tolerate slower work performance, the lack of interpersonal skills and the existence of poor attitudes toward work are often not countenanced, as they lead to conflict among staff, poor team performance, and refusal to follow instructions from supervisors. A survey of 175 business employers indicated that it was not specific vocational skills that improved an individual's employability, but the presence of positive work habits, the ability to follow basic instructions, and the ability to relate well to workmates (Wilms, 1984). Unfortunately, it is these very attributes that many TBI individuals lack.

Comprehensive programs that specifically target vocational rehabilitation are operating in the United States and Britain. The development of vocational rehabilitation programs reflected a growing recognition that the benefits of cognitive rehabilitation were not generalizing to work settings (Kreutzer et al., 1989). Vocational training programs were developed for inpatient settings where prevocational skills could be taught (e.g., communication skills, time management, personal hygiene) and TBI individuals could participate in simulated employment (e.g., work in the hospital cafeteria, or participation in an imaginary work setting that is created on the ward). Outpatient day programs and outpatient clinics also developed vocational rehabilitation programs that offered prevocational training and simulated employment, in addition to supervised work placements and planned reintegration into the TBI individual's preinjury work setting (e.g., Ben-Yishay et al., 1987b). A supported employment model has also been employed in which the TBI individual enters the workplace with a job coach who supervises his performance (Wehman et al., 1989b,c).

Uncontrolled studies have generally supported these models of vocational rehabilitation, as assessed by rates of return to employment (e.g., Rao et al., 1990). However, it is unclear from the research whether TBI individuals are working at the same level or being promoted at the same rate as they were prior to injury. In addition, many TBI individuals who were unemployed at the time of their injury remain unemployed. Whether these individuals would have obtained employment had they not been injured is not known.

In New Zealand, the vocational rehabilitation of TBI individuals is primarily the responsibility of the Accident Rehabilitation and Compensation Insurance Corporation (ARCIC). Throughout the country, the ARCIC employs client officers whose job it is to assist the TBI individuals' return to work by organizing work trials and work placements. Wages of TBI individuals are subsidized by the ARCIC until the return to work is as full as possible. Seven members of the family support program (i.e., 50%) successfully returned to work within 6 months of their injuries, without contact with ARCIC client officers. This result probably reflects the relatively mild nature of their TBI sequelae. Another three TBI individuals did not qualify for ARCIC vocational rehabilitation, as they were unemployed at the time of their accidents. The remaining four required ongoing assistance with vocational rehabilitation for more than 18 months after their accidents. These participants either failed to return to work or worked in a much reduced capacity. In these cases, vocational interventions were devised by the therapist and the client officer. The therapist was primarily responsible for coordinating the vocational rehabilitation of the participants in the family support program who were unemployed prior to their injuries.

Vocational Assessment

Successful work performance necessitates the application of a wide variety of skills. For instance, working on a construction site requires physical stamina to complete the lifting required, fast reaction time to be able to respond to danger, good short-term memory to remember verbal instructions, planning skills to formulate a sequence of actions to complete the building task, emotional stability to cope with the work pressure that arises as contractors strive to meet deadlines, interpersonal skills to be able to communicate with other workers, and motivation to keep working in an environment in which each worker has a degree of control over his pace of work. Because of the large number of skills that are required in a work setting, vocational assessment of the TBI individuals involved evaluating a wide range of areas, including preinjury work history, preinjury vocational skills, cognitive status, interpersonal skills, emotional functioning, physical functioning, behavioral difficulties, perceptual impairment, living skills, and fatiguability.

Completing this assessment involved a multidisciplinary approach whereby professionals from each discipline completed part of the assessment relevant to their professional competency (e.g., the physiotherapist assessed physical functioning, the speech language therapist assessed language/communication skills). Assessments were carried out utilizing observational assessment (e.g., skill level, work rate, and work quality), by interviewing the TBI individuals and their families, and by the use of questionnaires. Wehman et al. (1989a) have produced a "Consumer Screening Form" containing 28 questions that rehabilitation staff complete. The questions gather information on factors such as the TBI individual's strength, endurance, physical mobility, communication, social interaction skills, and motivation. Haffey and Lewis (1989) have also devised a very useful questionnaire they have titled "Barriers to Vocational Outcomes Profile." This measure lists 20 common barriers to successful return to work (e.g., social behavior, physical health) that are rated from 0 (no barrier) to 5 (unconditional barrier).

Following the completion of the vocational assessment, goals were set for each TBI individual. The goals stated in behavioral terms the desired outcome of the vocational rehabilitation program, whether this outcome was part-time work, full-time work, placement in a sheltered workshop, or a work trial. The family support program also employed the Haffey and Lewis (1989) concept of "essential events." Essential events are critical events that must occur if the vocational goals are to be met. For example, if a goal had been set for Peter to be able to work four days a week as a carpenter, essential events would include finding a job, enhancing his communication skills, and increasing his tolerance of frustration. All the essential events were written down and formed the basis of the vocational rehabilitation plan for the TBI individual.

Prevocational Training

Vocational assessments indicated that it was necessary for some TBI individuals to learn a variety of skills that were prerequisites to successful performance in the workplace. For example, Michael's vocational assessment indicated that he had extremely low tolerance for frustration and would be likely to be physically assaultive in the workplace. Thus, until Michael learned anger-management skills, he could not successfully cope with a work trial. Other TBI individuals needed to develop cognitive compensatory skills, communication skills, time-management skills, budgeting skills, and basic self-care skills (e.g., personal hygiene, dress). The teaching of such skills is referred to as "prevocational training" (Smith, 1983).

As attendance at work is totally reliant on the TBI individual's ability to maintain some form of structure within a day, the first priority for prevocational training was to assist TBI individuals to establish a daily routine that involved getting up at a regular time (e.g., 7:45 A.M.), eating at regular intervals, and scheduling activities during the day. This component of prevocational training was the responsibility of occupational therapists. Following the establishment of a daily routine, TBI individuals began a process that has been referred to as "work conditioning" (Gobble et al., 1987). Work conditioning involved increasing the TBI individuals' endurance by setting tasks designed to improve their physical and mental stamina. All TBI individuals were encouraged to exercise regularly and set goals for fitness that increased in difficulty over time. Keith, for example, swam twice a week for 3 weeks after discharge from the hospital. He then began to jog regularly and eventually began weight training. Simon (1988) provides an excellent example of work conditioning with a TBI individual whose goal was to return to work as a mechanic's assistant. The work conditioning program comprised tasks such as changing the oil in a vehicle, repairing a bicycle, changing an electrical socket, programming a video recorder, and changing the master brake cylinder on a car.

The TBI individual's progress was monitored during the prevocational phase, through regularly scheduled participation in simulated work activities. As the family support program was run on an outpatient basis, the simulated work activities involved a series of tasks set by the occupational therapist within the workshop (e.g., carrying out computer processing, constructing a cabinet, completing an accountancy task, cooking a meal). When a TBI individual had received 12–14 months of prevocational training and was still not ready for a work trial, a decision was made whether or not to consider a permanent placement in a sheltered workshop. The decision was made upon the basis of the TBI individual's degree of cognitive impairment, his motivation, the severity of his behavioral disturbances, and whether he had ever worked independently before his injuries (DePoy, 1987). Derek, for example, displayed severe cognitive impairment, had received prevocational training for over a year, had not succeeded at two work trials, and was poorly motivated to obtain employment. Hence, a decision was made that the most appropriate placement for Derek was in a sheltered workshop. Although initially reluctant to attend a sheltered workshop, Derek agreed when he recognized that attending the workshop would give him access to specialized woodworking machinery that he wanted to work with.

Vocational Placement

Following prevocational training, work placements were arranged for TBI individuals. Some TBI individuals returned to their preinjury workplace on the understanding that there was a permanent position available for them, either in their previous job or in a different capacity. Other TBI individuals were unable to return to their previous vocation due to the severity of their TBI sequelae (e.g., impaired language or cognitive ability). The ARCIC arranged vocational placements for these individuals. Under the ARCIC protocol, each TBI individual completed a variety of work placements until it was determined whether a permanent position could be found. Vocational placements lasted anywhere from 4 weeks to 18 months, and if successful could result in a permanent job.

Selecting an Appropriate Vocational Placement

The information gathered from the vocational assessment was used to determine the TBI individuals' existing skills and their ability to learn new skills. This information was combined with knowledge about the TBI individuals' preinjury vocational status and present interests, to select a vocational placement. Experience indicated that participants were more open to vocational placements that were either related to work they had done prior to their accident or in areas they had wanted to develop skills in. For example, Richard undertook a vocational placement as a freezing worker in a meat processing plant. Previously, he had worked as a laboratory technician in this setting. Some TBI individuals chose to retrain for a new vocation rather than return to their previous position in a lesser capacity (e.g., Justin attended college rather than work as a kitchen hand at the restaurant where he had previously been a chef).

In order to select an appropriate work placement, it was also necessary to evaluate the workplace and the nature of the tasks that the TBI individual was to carry out. This evaluation was generally the responsibility of the ARCIC client officer. This task-analysis process involved a step-by-step assessment of the skills necessary to complete each work task. A decision was made by the ARCIC client officer and the therapist in consultation with the TBI individual as to whether or not the individual would be able to learn how to complete each work task.

Preparing a TBI Individual and the Family for the Vocational Placement

When a vocational placement had been agreed upon, time was spent with the TBI individual and the family preparing them for the placement. Practical details such as transportation, the number of hours to be worked, and how the TBI individual would be paid were discussed. The family's participation in this process was critical, as it was the family who usually woke the TBI individual up in the morning, drove him to the workplace, and encouraged him to continue with the vocational placement when he became discouraged. If the family did not agree with the vocational placement (e.g., if they considered the job to be beneath the TBI individual), then there was always a possibility that they would not assist the TBI individual and would thereby essentially sabotage the work placement (Kreutzer et al., 1991).

The results of the task analysis were utilized to develop a list of instructions for the TBI individual about what needed to be done in order to complete the task. If the TBI individual's memory or planning ability was impaired, the steps in the task were written out as a checklist. In addition, the more difficult components of the task were rehearsed with the TBI individual (DePoy, 1987). Some individuals were also encouraged to write out a list of work rules (see also Kreutzer et al., 1991). For example, Hamish decided he was to spend no more than 3 hours a day on bookwork (e.g., doing accounts or studying), would take a long lunch break, and would ask workmates to assist him with computer programming.

Educating the Employer

Typically, employers were unaware of the long-term impact that TBI can have on work performance. While they appeared to realize that difficulties with memory and motivation were normal following TBI, their expectation was for these difficulties to improve to preinjury levels approximately 2 months after the vocational placement begun. This expectation for rapid recovery meant that they initially assigned light duties, then progressively more difficult tasks over time. Generally, in the early phases of returning to work, the TBI individuals coped very well, and ARCIC services were often withdrawn. However, approximately 4 months later, when the work demands were increased, significant problems in the TBI individuals' ability to cope at work often became apparent. This situation left employers seriously dissatisfied with the TBI individuals' job performance.

Peter's employer, for example, wanted him to leave his job because of his poor performance 6 months after his accident. However, when education regarding the long-term nature of vocational readjustment following TBI was provided, the employer was happy to delay making a decision about Peter's employability for another 6 months. In general, the employers appreciated the opportunity to discuss the TBI individuals' work performance. Employers also expressed considerable relief at the offer of assistance from the therapist should the TBI individual develop any work-related difficulties.

Monitoring the Vocational Placement

Once vocational placements had commenced, the TBI individuals' progress was closely monitored. The ARCIC client officer made regular on-site visits, phoned employers, and met with the TBI individuals to discuss their performance. Both employers and TBI individuals were questioned about the TBI individuals' punctuality, appearance, ability to work independently, work productivity, quality of work, and interpersonal relationships with supervisors and workmates. Wehman et al. (1989c) provide a useful 10-question employer/supervisor rating scale that assesses work speed, attendance, communication, and consistency of performance. Employers rate their satisfaction with these aspects of work performance on a scale from 1 (extreme dissatisfaction) to 5 (extreme satisfaction). The benefit of this scale is that it requires little effort to complete and can provide a baseline for assessing change in the TBI individual's performance over time.

Clear feedback was given to the TBI individuals regarding their work performance. In most cases, it was necessary to assist employers to give feedback, as the provision of feedback of this nature was not a usual practice within the many work settings. During the monitoring phase, skills training also took place utilizing behavioral techniques (e.g., teaching successive approximations, repeated practice, rewarding for adequate quality of work) and compensatory strategies (e.g., the use of diaries, mnemonic techniques). The therapist also monitored the TBI individuals to ensure that their participation in the vocational placement did not adversely affect other areas of their life. For example, Keith's substance abuse worsened when he began a paid vocational placement, as he had additional funds to buy drugs. Other families reported increases in the TBI individual's fatigue and irritability once a vocational placement commenced. When problems such as these were identified, appropriate interventions were made (e.g., direct credit of wages to a savings account, reduction in number of work hours).

Work Evaluation

Occasionally, vocational placements were not successful. Derek, for example, consistently failed to show up at his workplace. When he did show up, his supervisor reported that he was unmotivated and unable to work without close supervision. Richard had similar problems in that his attendance at his vocational placement was sporadic. Furthermore, he frequently arrived late and left early without completing any work. In situations in which work trials were not successful, work evaluations were requested by ARCIC rehabilitation officers to ensure that emotional disturbance and cognitive impairment were not affecting the TBI individual's work performance. Work evaluations involved careful assessment of the individual and his work environment. A range of factors were considered, including the level of supervision the TBI individual was receiving from employers, whether the TBI individual had the necessary skills to successfully complete the work, and whether emotional disturbance was impacting the TBI individual's work performance.

Derek's work evaluation, for instance, revealed that the work environment was a major contributor to the difficulties he was experiencing. He was actually receiving very little supervision, no feedback was given to him regarding his work performance, and he had not been given the opportunity to learn any new skills. These deficiencies resulted in boredom and erratic work attendance. In contrast to Derek's situation, Richard's work environment was excellent, but he was having difficulty working in a setting that he associated with his friend who had died in the accident. Additionally, Richard's cognitive impairment resulted in his being unable to concentrate for even short periods of time and becoming rapidly fatigued.

The information gained from work evaluations was used to make recommendations for improving the TBI individuals' work performance. Gradual reintroduction to the workplace (e.g., moving from part-time work once a week to part-time work three times a week), guided practice, extra tuition, and graduated reintroduction to difficult work tasks were the most frequent recommendations. In some cases, a change to a more appropriate work environment was recommended (e.g., Derek moved to a sheltered workshop environment), or suggestions were made with the aim of improving the work environments. TBI individuals frequently needed new equipment to improve the quality of their performance (e.g., replacing a typewriter with a word processor) or relocation from a noisy room to a quieter work area. Recommended areas for assessing work placements are as follows:

1. *Is the work environment appropriate*? For example, is there loud noise that may be distracting to the TBI individual? Is the equipment in the workplace stored in an orderly manner?
2. *Is the task appropriate*? For example, is the work too easy for the TBI individual? Does the TBI individual have specific impairments (e.g., profound memory deficits) that prevent successful completion of the task?
3. *Is the TBI individual implementing compensatory strategies*? For example, is the TBI individual using a diary to note down the jobs he is expected to complete?

4. *Is adequate supervision being provided*? For example, is the TBI individual receiving clear feedback on his performance? Is on-the-job training being provided? Does the TBI individual have a supervisor to whom he is responsible?
5. *Are there psychological factors impacting the TBI individual's work performance*? For example, is there any indication that the TBI individual is depressed?
6. *Are the employer's expectations realistic*? For example, does the employer expect the TBI individual to be performing at the same level as he was prior to the injury?

Vocational Counseling

The major obstacle faced by TBI individuals in attempting to return to employment was their difficulty in acknowledging the reductions in their ability and their refusal to readjust their expectations regarding their work performance. Indeed, as Ben-Yishay et al. (1987b) comment, poor self-awareness and unrealistic expectations are the primary contributors to poor vocational adjustment. As work performance was a primary source of self-worth for many of the participants, reduced ability to work presented a major threat to their self-esteem. In order to bolster their self-esteem, participants tended to overestimate their skills and request vocational placements that they were unable to complete successfully. Considerable time was spent helping the TBI individuals reevaluate what a realistic work expectation for them was. This process was most challenging for TBI individuals who had held positions of considerable responsibility prior to their injuries and who had sustained severe disability postinjury (see also Kreutzer et al., 1991). When the TBI individual was not able to readjust to his former work station, finding an acceptable vocational placement was very difficult and depressed mood frequently resulted. For example, Graham frequently became depressed when he failed to complete as much work in a day as he had prior to his accident. Eventually, an alternative vocational placement had to be established in which Graham had no preinjury work experience against which to judge his performance and decide he had not completed an adequate amount of work.

AMELIORATING BEHAVIORAL DISORDERS

Behavioral disorders are common following TBI (e.g., Elsass & Kinsella, 1987; Godfrey et al., 1993a). The literature is replete with case examples of TBI individuals who spit (Wood, 1987), swear (Burke & Lewis, 1986), are physically aggressive (Turner et al., 1990), shout (Alderman, 1991), are unable to complete self-care tasks (Tate, 1987a,b), and have very low levels of goal-directed activity.

Behaviors such as these present formidable barriers to the resumption of preinjury social roles in the occupational, interpersonal, and family domains (Haffey & Scibak, 1989; Zahara & Cuvo, 1984). Consequently, it is essential to ameliorate behavioral disorders if social roles are to be successfully maintained following TBI.

To date, the more extreme behavioral disorders (e.g., severe physical aggression toward others) have been managed using stringent behavior modification procedures carried out in specialized inpatient rehabilitation units (Wood, 1988b). These methods may be justified in cases of serious behavioral disorder, but were considered too restrictive for TBI individuals in the family support program who presented with less severe problems such as impulsivity, low motivation, and aggression. Accordingly, a more educative approach employing less stringent behavior modification techniques in combination with cognitive strategies was applied within the context of the TBI individuals' everyday environment (e.g., their home or workplace).

Reducing Behavioral Excesses

The intervention approach for reducing behavioral excesses comprised five principal techniques that are described below. These strategies were used for a wide variety of behavioral excesses such as shouting, swearing, and physical aggression.

Education

Education was provided to ensure that both the TBI individuals and their families were aware that behavioral excesses are a "normal" problem following TBI. It was emphasized that the occurrence of behavioral problems reflected neither the TBI individual's "being impossible" nor the family's "failure to cope." In addition to the standard education program, a very helpful manual by DeBoskey and Morin (1985) was given to families when appropriate. This manual outlines a number of excellent guidelines for dealing with behavioral problems such as swearing, verbal outbursts, and temper tantrums. In some cases, the families were able to successfully implement the recommended guidelines without any assistance from the therapist.

Antecedent Control Techniques

When a "trigger" for the behavioral excess was identified, antecedent control techniques (Zencius, Wesolowski, Burke, & McQuade, 1989) were put in place. For example, Justin would yell and shout insulting comments at his partner each time she failed to respond to his requests instantly. Similarly, Peter would have a verbal outburst at his brother, followed by door slamming and social withdrawal, when they disagreed in a discussion. Aaron would invariably swear and make inappropriate comments (e.g., "I'm going to rape Mrs. X") when he was very fatigued or when he felt threatened by the content of a conversation and wanted to change the topic. It was explained to the TBI individuals and their families that these situations are like green traffic lights, in that they are consistently responded to in the same way, the behavior being largely automatic.

TBI individuals and their families were advised to avoid the trigger situations when possible (e.g., when Aaron was tired, he would go to sleep rather than talk to his family). Alternatively, the TBI individual could be distracted in the trigger situation by a family member's asking him to engage in another activity. Prompts were also used to remind the TBI individual to be careful in trigger situations. For instance, Justin had a note in his diary that prompted him to be patient and helpful when he arrived home. Families found it useful to present potentially upsetting information to the TBI individual in a neutral manner. Hearing that "the hospital says driving is not advisable until later" provokes a far milder response than "You're not a good driver" or "Your father says you can't." The antecedent control techniques were most effective when combined with contingency management.

Contingency Management

Contingency management techniques were employed both to increase the frequency of adaptive behavioral responding and to reduce the frequency and severity of behavioral problems. Social reinforcement (i.e., praise, attention) was provided by the therapist, or the family, or both, when the TBI individual coped with difficult situations appropriately. Aaron, for instance, was complimented each time he used his kick bag or played music when he was angry. Prior to this, he had lashed out verbally at whoever was near him at the time. Families were also encouraged not to inadvertently reinforce behavioral excesses by "giving in" to the TBI individuals' demands or by allowing them to avoid certain tasks. Derek, for instance, became restless and would wander around the house making sarcastic comments whenever his partner spent time with her children. Initially, his partner had responded by turning her attention to Derek. Unfortunately, this response produced an increase in the frequency of his sarcastic comments and restless behavior. A contingency management stratagem was instituted whereby she would ignore his restless behavior and continue to spend time with the children. Because the reinforcer for Derek's behavior was actually spending time with his partner, it was also decided to establish a period each day during which they were alone together. This plan proved to be highly successful, and Derek's sarcastic comments and restless behavior soon decreased in frequency. His partner also benefitted by being able to spend uninterrupted time with her children.

Family members were encouraged to respond calmly when the TBI individual behaved inappropriately. This prevented inadvertent reinforcement of these behavioral excesses. Aaron's father, for instance, had suffered a stroke and had difficulty controlling his reactions to Aaron's disinhibited speech. On one occasion, he became extremely angry with Aaron, and while yelling at him he backed him against a wall. Aaron responded by putting his fist through the wall. In circumstances like these, the relative involved was advised to leave the primary care of the TBI individual to another family member and focus instead on spending short periods of time engaging in pleasant activities with the TBI individual. Whenever possible, the therapist modeled more appropriate ways of responding to inappropriate behavior. For example, when TBI participants became sexually explicit during family education sessions, the therapist would calmly pay no attention to the explicit language and would change the topic. Later, the therapist would give feedback to the TBI individual about the behavior and what effect it had and would describe more appropriate behavior for that situation. The therapist's demonstration of responding calmly, ignoring behavioral excesses, and redirecting the TBI individual provided the family with a model of how such situations could be handled.

In cases in which inappropriate behavior was a frequent occurrence, a "how to handle" plan was written down, after consultation between the TBI individual and the family. Derek and his partner drew up a plan for handling situations in which he became angry and verbally abusive. They agreed that when he became angry, he was to go immediately to his room and write down what was annoying him. He would then choose a relaxing activity from a list he had compiled. Kate would ignore his behavior and, if this had no effect, remind him about the agreed-upon plan. She also had the option of calling on the assistance of Derek's brother if the situation worsened. Role-playing scenarios in which Derek became angry and plan implementation was practiced assisted Derek and his family to cope with the behavior in the agreed manner. The plan helped both parties deal with what was a very difficult behavioral problem.

Cognitive Strategies

Cognitive strategies designed to ameliorate behavioral excesses such as swearing or impulse behavior were taught to both the TBI individuals and their families. The main cognitive strategy employed to reduce behavioral excesses was cognitive reappraisal. In cognitive reappraisal, the participants sat down and reevaluated the situation by thinking through what had happened. For example, if the TBI individuals had become angry, they were encouraged to think about whether they had understood the situation properly. A good illustration of this process is provided by its application with Peter. Peter repeatedly became extremely angry with his family when they tried to help him, as he interpreted this assistance to mean that he was inadequate. However, when he reconsidered the situation and recognized that most TBI individuals need help in the early phases of recovery, his outbursts abated and he accepted the assistance graciously.

Skills Training

Several participants displayed quite impulsive behavior patterns. Susan, for example, put her hand straight through a window to reach the door latch when she found herself locked out of her house. Similarly, when Keith found that he disliked the boarders he had living with him, he sold his house within the week and moved in with his parents. Most behavioral excesses following TBI are in fact purposeful and goal-directed, aimed at either obtaining reinforcement or avoiding or escaping aversive stimuli (Haffey & Scibak, 1989). Given the goal-directed nature of this behavior, it is important to teach TBI individuals the skills necessary to achieve their goals in a more appropriate manner. Once the TBI individuals were able to gain attention in an appropriate manner, communicate more appropriately about what annoyed them, or formulate a strategy to enable them to successfully carry out a task, they became less likely to yell, behave impulsively, and throw things. For this reason, assertiveness skills, communication skills, and problem-solving skills were taught to the TBI individuals.

Summary of the Procedure for Reducing Behavioral Excesses

1. Educate the TBI individual and his family regarding the type of behavioral problems that result from TBI.
2. Provide the family with self-help books outlining management strategies.
3. Teach the TBI individual and his family how to identify "trigger" situations and how to avoid them.
4. Encourage the family to give social reinforcement when the TBI individual uses appropriate coping strategies.
5. Encourage the family not to acquiesce if the TBI individual behaves in an unreasonable manner.
6. Act as a real-life model to demonstrate to families how to use management strategies (e.g., ignoring behavioral excesses, redirecting the TBI individual to an alternative activity).
7. Provide feedback to the TBI individual about why certain behaviors are appropriate, and describe appropriate alternative behaviors.
8. Ask the TBI individual and his family to write a "how to handle" plan together. Encourage the TBI individual and his family to role play a problematic situation (e.g., when the TBI individual is angry), and ask them to demonstrate how they would implement the "how to handle" plan.

9. Teach the TBI individual and his family appropriate skills that serve the same function as the inappropriate behavior (e.g., communication skills, assertiveness training).
10. Encourage the TBI individual and his family to reappraise problematic situations (e.g., change appraisals from "They are being difficult" to "What do I need to do to cope with this?").

Decreasing Addictive Behaviors

Another category of excessive behavior addressed within the family support program was that of addiction. According to Langley, Lindsay, Lam, and Priddy (1990), the dual problem of substance abuse and traumatic brain injury is well recognized by rehabilitation workers. All participants in our study were screened for the presence of preinjury substance abuse; however, only one individual, Keith, acknowledged any significant substance abuse problem. Because of the potential harmful effects of continued substance abuse, Keith decided to abstain from alcohol following his TBI, and an intervention plan was instituted to help him achieve this goal. This intervention was based upon the procedure of Langley et al. (1990) and involved reviewing the negative consequences alcohol consumption had on Keith's life (e.g., drunk driving charges, financial problems), providing education regarding the effects of alcohol, and avoiding situations that were associated with a high probability of drinking (e.g., going to a bar). In addition, activities were scheduled to help distract Keith from thinking about alcohol, and Keith asked his friends to encourage him not to drink. A relapse-prevention program was also implemented as described by Marlatt and Gordon (1985). At 22 months after his injury, Keith remained abstinent and had regained his driving license, which had been revoked for over 14 years as a result of drunk driving convictions. His abstinence from alcohol was confirmed by his mother, with whom he had close contact. However, there was evidence that his cannabis use increased at the time he decreased his alcohol intake.

One participant developed a gambling problem following his TBI. When Richard found that he was unable to tolerate alcohol, he felt uncomfortable drinking nonalcoholic beverages while sitting in a bar. Unfortunately, the bar was his main source of social contact. His alternative behavior to drinking was to play the poker machines that were in the same room. This gambling quickly developed into a serious problem, and within 3 weeks he was spending amounts ranging from \$45 to \$65 daily. He immediately put any winnings back into the poker machine, which resulted in further financial losses.

Initially, education was provided about problem gambling and how it is maintained by intermittent reinforcement. Richard was unconvinced of this explanation. Therefore, he was advised to keep a record of the amount of money he spent and the amount of money he won. Record keeping demonstrated to him that he was not in fact winning as much money as he had thought. Goals for controlled gambling were set (Rankin, 1982). Each week, Richard set a limit on the amount of money he could spend on gambling. The amount was decreased each week by approximately $10. This procedure met with moderate success (see days 5–19 in Figure 5.2). However, Richard decided he was still gambling too much, at which point the number of days he was allowed to visit the bar was also restricted. Restrictions resulted in even further reductions in spending (see days 20–35 in Figure 5.2). His social contact at this time also increased as a result of attending a training course, which provided him with an alternative source of social contact. Follow-up 8 weeks later revealed that his gambling behavior had all but ceased.

Assisting Families to Implement Behavior Management Programs

The implementation of behavioral programs can be very demanding for families. In the early phases following injury, families tend to tolerate behavioral disturbances and explain them away (Tate, 1987b). Consequently, when a behavioral program is suggested, the family is faced with changing their almost automatic responses to the TBI individual's behavior (e.g., habitually giving the TBI individual what he wants to prevent shouting). To be successful, behavioral programs require monitoring of and consistent response to the TBI individual's

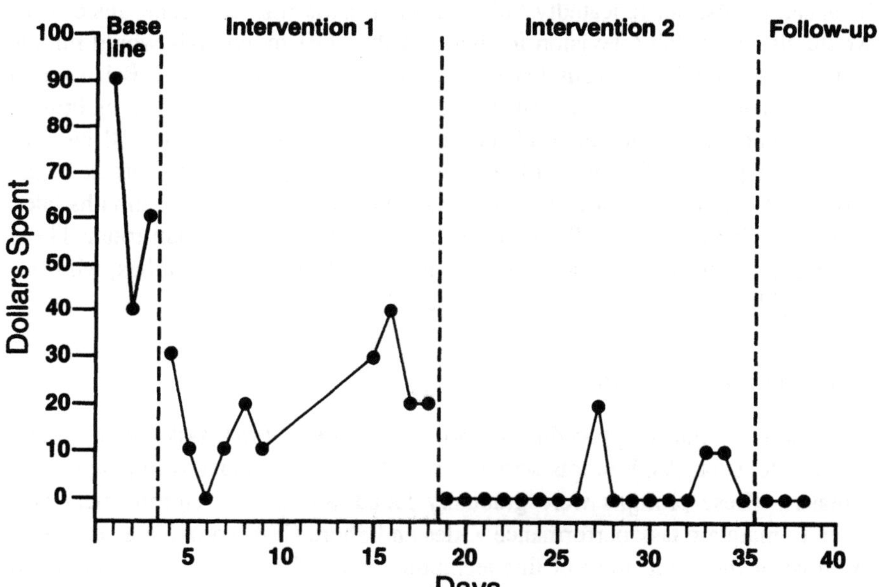

FIGURE 5.2. Money spent on gambling.

behavior. The families in the support program had some difficulty meeting the requirements of consistency and monitoring, as they were usually very busy and were often struggling to cope with their own emotional reactions to their difficult circumstances. For these reasons, behavioral techniques needed to be applied in a flexible manner. Flexibility was achieved by strategies such as restricting the amount of record keeping to a minimum, asking different family members and friends to take responsibility for the behavioral program each week, and ensuring that the interventions were designed to take into account the restrictions that TBI individuals and their families faced (e.g., limited free time, motivational difficulties). Making these adaptations to behavioral programs resulted in interventions that were easier for families to implement.

Managing Behavioral Deficits

The presence of behavioral deficits in TBI individuals has been well documented (e.g., Wood, 1987). Behavioral deficits refer to appropriate behavior that occurs at low frequency (e.g., taking medication, showering). Behavioral deficits are hypothesized to result from brain-stem and cortical damage that reduces the TBI individual's level of general arousal (Wood & Burgess, 1988). The behavioral deficits displayed by the TBI individuals in the family support program were not lack of self-care skills (e.g., cooking, hygiene), but rather a persistent difficulty in initiating and completing tasks. Derek was able to shower, shave, and prepare balanced meals, but repeatedly failed to do so if he was left alone. Instead, he would sit and watch television for hours. Other TBI individuals would initiate activity only after being prompted to do so by a relative. For example, Brian would leave his laundry on the floor until his father had repeatedly prompted him. Prior to his accident, Brian completed this chore without prompting. Some TBI individuals began jobs readily but took a long time to complete them. Patrick began tidying up his garden, but had not completed the task more than 6 months later. Likewise, Grant took over 9 months to finish wallpapering a small room. These experiences were frustrating to the TBI individuals and their families, who frequently felt that nothing was being achieved.

Task-Analysis Procedure

The task-analysis procedure involved three steps. First, tasks were broken into smaller subtasks. Prompts were given to the TBI individual to complete these subtasks. These prompts were gradually faded, and social reinforcement was given to maintain task performance. Giles and Shore (1989) provide a very good example of the application of this technique with a 20-year-old TBI individual who was neither washing nor dressing. A 16-step program was devised, and the TBI individual was given prompts to complete each step of the program. If any of the steps were completed without a prompt being supplied, the TBI individual was praised. The TBI individual also verbally rehearsed the procedure during the day in order to facilitate task learning.

Goal Setting and Contingency Management

Goal setting and contingency management proved to be the most successful methods for increasing goal-directed activity. Derek, for instance, greatly increased his initiation of activity when he set and completed four goals each week (e.g., clean up bedroom, buy a shirt, vacuum the lounge), and Brian's tendency to not wash his dirty clothes changed rapidly once his father ceased prompting him and left the laundry on his bedroom floor. Brian then quickly discovered the negative consequences of not doing laundry (i.e., dirty socks and no clean work shirts) and began to regularly wash his clothes. Similarly, Derek agreed that he was to listen to music only after he had completed his diary. Within one week, his daily diary completion rate rose to 100%.

Intervention Effectiveness

Unfortunately, regardless of the intervention technique employed, the degree of maintenance and generalization of gains was limited. The frequency of targeted activities would usually increase; however, activity levels in other areas often remained static. For example, at the completion of the program, Brian was still doing his own laundry, but he also continued to spend most of his free time sitting down apparently doing nothing and failing to communicate with other family members. These interventions produced results similar to those reported by others who have found that behavioral deficits have a poor prognosis (e.g., Wood & Burgess, 1988).

IMPLEMENTING INTERVENTIONS TO IMPROVE SOCIAL COMPETENCY

Social competency encompasses a diverse variety of skills (e.g., communication skills, self-monitoring skills) that are relevant to all social roles (e.g., occupation, leisure, and friendships). Careful assessment is necessary to ensure that interventions are chosen that accurately target the underlying problem. For example, implementing an interpersonal-skills training program for a TBI individual with few friends will not be effective if the underlying problem is the TBI individual's poor motivation. Interventions also need to be appropriate to the TBI individual's ability level. Thus, for TBI individuals who display severe global cognitive impairment, the use of behavioral interventions to teach basic skills (e.g., hygiene routines) may be more appropriate. For TBI individuals with more intact cognitive abilities, conversational-skills training might be a more appropriate intervention.

TBI individuals need to be coached at least twice weekly if skills training is to be effective. If this is not possible, family members or friends need to be taught how to practice the skills with the TBI individuals, and practice sessions need to be scheduled. Without appropriate training, skills tend to be forgotten or to fail to be generalized from one setting (e.g., home) to another setting (e.g., workplace). Finally, it is necessary to stress the importance of preventative interventions such as education, goal setting, ongoing monitoring, and prompting. If these interventions are applied early enough, the deterioration of social networks, decline in leisure activities, and failure of vocational placements can be prevented.

6

Fostering Family Adaptation

Families face a myriad of adverse changes in role functioning, financial status, and expectations for their future following traumatic brain injury (TBI) to a family member. The impact of these changes is frequently depression, anxiety, anger, and guilt (Lezak, 1978; Livingston et al., 1985a,b; Shaw & McMahon, 1990), with some research going so far as to suggest that family members may become even more burdened than the individual who has been injured (Brooks, 1991). Burden escalates over time and is associated with the severity of the TBI individual's cognitive and social problems (Livingston, 1985b; Oddy et al., 1978a). Family burden also tends to be chronic. For example, Brooks (1991) reports that 89% of the relatives he studied reported medium to high levels of subjective burden 5 years following the occurrence of the injury.

Because of the adverse impact TBI has upon families, there is general recognition of the need to offer services to families (e.g., J. R. Johnson & Higgins, 1987; Prigatano et al., 1986a). It is necessary to support families not only to bolster the psychological well-being of family members, but also to enhance the beneficial impact the family may have upon the TBI member's adjustment. For example, having a supportive family available is associated with faster rehabilitative progress for the injured member (Mauss-Clum & Ryan, 1981). Rehabilitation workers also rely upon families to provide much of the information that is necessary to assess problems and the effectiveness of interventions (McKinlay & Hickox, 1988). However, despite these proclamations of the need to involve families, very little specific detail about how to support families has been published (Shaw & McMahon, 1990). Hence, one of the major aims of the family support program was to develop and empirically evaluate an intervention program for families that could be replicated by other workers in the field. The strategies utilized in the program to support families are outlined in this chapter.

PROVIDING FAMILIES WITH INFORMATION

Families frequently express a need for detailed information about TBI and its long-term effects (Mauss-Clum & Ryan, 1981; Panting & Merry, 1972). In more recent times, this need has been acknowledged, and a variety of education programs have been developed (e.g., Rosenthal, 1984). The rationale for educating families is that providing information will minimize fear of the unknown (Grinspun, 1987), increase cooperation with health care workers, and, most important, improve the family's ability to cope with the injured member's behavior (J. R. Johnson & Higgins, 1987). Unfortunately, difficulties in implementing family education programs are not uncommon. For example, families may not retain information because of their high level of distress (Mauss-Clum & Ryan, 1981), may not accept the validity of information given (Sanguinetti & Catanzaro, 1987), and may fail to attend education sessions (Rao et al., 1986). The education module developed for the family support program was designed to overcome some of these problems. This module is described in the following sections. Excerpts from education sessions with Graham and his family will be used to illustrate the techniques employed during family education sessions.

Content

The education module utilized in the family support program comprised four sessions that were held at weekly intervals. Each session addressed topics such as the nature of traumatic brain injury, outcome after traumatic brain injury, and ways of coping with the difficulties that may arise following TBI. Written summaries were prepared for each topic (see Appendix A), which contained relevant New Zealand research findings on TBI. Any additional information that was requested by the family but not included in the module was provided within 7 days after the request was made. A variety of such requests were made for information on topics ranging from posttraumatic epilepsy to pain management to use of alcohol and cannabis.

Participation

Clinical experience has indicated that siblings, and sometimes parents, are reluctant to involve themselves in education sessions held at outpatient clinics (see also Sherr & Langenbahn, 1992). This reluctance can arise for a number of reasons. Many people feel awkward when they enter hospital settings. Often, family members have taken considerable time off work while the TBI individual was in the hospital and are unable to arrange further leave. If families do attend hospital appointments, siblings and children rarely come, and often a single family representative (e.g., the mother or wife) will accompany the TBI member.

In view of families' reluctance to attend hospital-based education programs, it was necessary to implement innovative strategies to increase their participation in education. One method of increasing participation was to hold education sessions in the evenings at the TBI individual's home, which allowed friends, parents, siblings, and children to attend with the minimum of inconvenience. During the family support program, each evening education session was attended by approximately three to five people. This was a greater number on average than had ever attended the education sessions that prior to the family support program had been offered in the clinic setting.

Timing

The timing of family education is an important consideration. Information regarding brain injury is typically presented to TBI victims and their families during the hospitalization phase (e.g., Grinspun, 1987; Rao et al., 1986; Sanguinetti & Catanzaro, 1987). Unfortunately, the patient and the family frequently fail to assimilate the information at this time because the patient's short-term memory is often poor and the family is as yet unaware of the problems that will arise when the patient returns home. In the earliest stages of recovery, families also tend to focus exclusively on the physical recovery and may be unwilling or unable to accept the information about the long-term psychosocial sequelae of TBI. Certainly, many of the TBI individuals and families in the support program could not recall the information about TBI that had been given to them during the hospitalization period. An excerpt from a transcript of a family education session demonstrates these problems:

Therapist: How much did they actually tell you when you were in the hospital?
TBI individual: Nothing that I remember.
Family member: Very scattered. I didn't know what questions to ask.

Because of these difficulties in offering education during the hospitalization phase, the education module was not offered until at least 3 months after injury. However, during the hospitalization phase, participants were given a basic education handout, and their questions were answered by hospital staff.

Method of Delivery

All information in the education module was presented in both verbal and written forms. Aids such as three-dimensional models of the brain were utilized, and time was spent personalizing the information by considering the results of the TBI individual's X rays, computed tomography (CT) scans, and neuropsychological test results. When possible, visual illustrations of the information being presented were provided. For example, coup and contracoup damage was demonstrated by placing a tennis ball in a large jar of water and tapping the jar forcefully on one side. The tennis ball hits one side of the jar and bounces back to hit the side directly opposite, demonstrating the coup–contracoup effect. Such visual illustrations greatly enhanced the participants' understanding of the information that was presented.

Education sessions were carried out in an interactive format, with over half the time being spent in discussion rather than the didactic presentation of information. Equal emphasis was placed upon addressing issues of concern to the family members and the TBI individual. During the education sessions, role plays were instigated (e.g., what would the family member say to the TBI individual when the individual requested to use the car?), goals were set, and every attempt was made to apply the information to the individual's own situation (e.g., what memory aids would be best for his use?). All participants were encouraged to ask questions, with many families finding it helpful to note questions between sessions so that they could be brought up at the next session. In some cases, education sessions were tape recorded so that the family could refer back to them.

Summary of the Procedure for Education Modules

1. Schedule the education module for several weeks after the TBI individual has been discharged from the hospital.
2. Obtain the results of CT scans, X rays, and neuropsychological testing, and discuss these findings with the family.
3. Ensure that education is provided in an interactive discussion format, with equal attention being paid to the TBI individual and to the family members.
4. Provide written summaries of the education material.
5. Use visual demonstrations to illustrate the information that is being presented (e.g., use three-dimensional models of the brain).
6. Consider taping the sessions for the family's future reference.
7. Hold the education sessions at a time (e.g., after work hours) and in a place (e.g., in the home) that is convenient for the family.
8. Inform families that education is offered to all families and is not an indication that health professionals think the family is not coping.

Gaining Entry and Building Rapport

Education sessions served not only as a way to present information about TBI, but also as a forum for a variety of other therapeutic activities. For example, some families and TBI individuals initially refused rehabilitation services because they perceived TBI to be a short-term problem that would end soon after the patient was discharged from the hospital. Other families refused services because they felt that accepting help was equivalent to acknowledging that there were problems that they were failing to cope with. In such cases, offering a "standard education module" was an excellent method of gaining entry into the family. The standard education module was offered to all families regardless of whether they were experiencing problems or not and regardless of whether they were coping or not. During the "standard education module," rapport was built through listening carefully to the individual and family, identifying the issues that were of importance to them, and empathizing with their feelings. Later, when difficulties became evident, the family had access to someone whom they knew and trusted to contact for help. It was common in the family support program for the family to agree reluctantly to a "standard education module" and then quickly recontact the health professional when problems arose.

Education and Emotional Expression

Education sessions provided family members with the opportunity to express how they had felt during the early phases of the TBI member's hospitalization. Often, family members had not had a chance to speak about this, nor had the TBI member had the opportunity to view his accident from the family's perspective. Hearing the family members' version of events was often invaluable for the TBI member, who could then better understand that traumatic brain injury affected not just him but the whole family. Moreover, support and encouragement could be offered to family members who had themselves experienced a very traumatic ordeal. The excerpt below is from Graham's first education session, in which the therapist discusses with the family the sequence of events surrounding the accident. According to Graham's family members, this was the first occasion on which Graham had acknowledged the impact that his accident had upon his family.

Family member: He didn't really come out of that coma for a couple of days, so I thought it was quite serious . . . actually not knowing was hard . . .

Therapist: It must have been difficult just sitting and waiting.

Family member: . . . they were helpful to an extent, but it was dreadful. You didn't know what was going to happen, if he was going to die . . . if it might mean he would still recover.

Therapist: It's the uncertainty of it all.

Family member: Yes, it's so emotional too.

TBI individual: Imagine the horror of being on the other side of the bed.

Assessment

During education sessions, a number of assessment tasks were carried out. For example, injury severity was verified (e.g., posttraumatic amnesia), premorbid adjustment was documented, and impairments were assessed. The education material contained lists of possible TBI effects. Participants were asked which, if any, of these effects they had experienced. Asking participants to identify the problems they had encountered on such a list often resulted in the identification of difficulties that had not previously been acknowledged through direct questioning. The education sessions had the added advantage that both the individual with the brain injury and most of the family members were present to corroborate details.

Therapist: Are you having any trouble remembering things like what time meetings are or people's names?

TBI individual: Not so much lately, but I definitely used to.

Therapist: [refers question to family member by gesture]

Family member: Definitely yes . . . he is a good actor. For a long time, I actually thought he was quite good . . . he was trying not to show he couldn't remember.

TBI individual: . . . young [could not remember the person's name] that works with my father . . . he would come in and say, "Good day, how are things with you," and he knew I didn't know his name.

Raising Awareness through Feedback

The education sessions provided a relatively nonthreatening setting in which feedback could be delivered to the TBI individual both by the family members and by the therapist. The TBI client found it easier to accept feedback in the context of an education session than in a one-on-one therapy session. The following excerpt is from an education session on social-skills deficits following TBI. The TBI individual involved had a tendency to talk at length on subjects that were not of interest to his listeners. His family found his overtalkativeness irritating, but had not told him about it for fear of hurting his feelings. In this session, both the therapist and the family were able to provide the TBI client with specific feedback concerning his social skills.

TBI individual: I don't feel I need to be too concerned about this [i.e., social skills].

Therapist: Your voice modulation is fine, your eye contact is fine . . . the one thing that you have pinpointed before is perhaps the talking and the length of time on your talking. [Family member's name], what do you think about this?

Family member: . . . he's having trouble there. . . .

In situations in which insightful statements were made by the TBI person or a family member, such statements were reinforced by the therapist (e.g., "It's good that you have noticed that"), and the person was encouraged to expand upon what he or she had said. In this way, from the very early sessions onwards, realistic expectations and accurate self-appraisal were promoted. In the following excerpt, the therapist has just explained that if unrealistically high expectations about work performance are held, then greater frustration is likely to result when goals are not met.

TBI individual: . . . I think I've always had great expectations on some things . . . I've lost this now to a degree and that annoys me . . . I'm prepared to take longer now . . . I was just saying today give it a bit more time . . .

Therapist: What's the worst thing about having your expectations changed?

TBI individual: You've got to motivate yourself and do something else. It's sometimes hard to find what else to have a go at. It's definitely going to take a little longer, but all I can still see is myself as a [occupation before the traumatic brain injury] . . .

Therapist: You're dead right it will take a bit longer, but if you know it's going to take a few years, you are less likely to be distressed.

TBI individual: Definitely.

Reinforcing Coping

The education sessions also provided an excellent opportunity to sincerely reinforce families and TBI individuals for coping well. Most families praised the TBI member for his efforts to adjust, but failed to recognize how well they themselves had adapted to extremely trying circumstances. Therefore, every opportunity was taken to reinforce the fact that problems such as arguments and anger outbursts are common following TBI and that despite the problems, the family had done a good job of supporting the TBI member. The reinforcing comments served to give a sense of hope to family members. Where possible, the therapist also pinpointed the specific aspects of coping that were adaptive. In the excerpt below, the therapist reinforces both the TBI individual and the family member for how well they are coping with the TBI sequelae.

Family member: Yes, I feel that [TBI individual's name] needs reassurance . . .

TBI individual: I'm lacking confidence in a lot of things.

Therapist: . . . you both need to know that you are doing well. I can honestly tell you that you are both doing a marvelous job. I am thrilled about things like [family member's name] not naming things for you [TBI individual had word-finding impairment] and with you having realistic expectations about getting back to work and not saying you can do the things that you are no longer able to do.

PROMOTING HEALTHY FAMILY RELATIONSHIPS

Marriage and Other Partnerships

For a number of reasons, relationship counseling is often necessary following TBI. The partners of TBI patients may struggle with loneliness when affectional and sexual needs are not met (Lezak, 1978). While other people may turn to their partners for reassurance during a crisis, TBI victims are frequently responsible for the crises and are not able to support or communicate with their partners. Partners of TBI individuals report lessened consensus, expression, and sense of personal reward in their relationships (L. C. Peters et al., 1992b). Frequently, partners describe feeling deserted by relatives, at the very time when they are being required to change from the role of a partner to the role of a caregiver. Even if the TBI individual does improve and return to competitive work, partners may constantly worry about their safety. Not surprisingly, the divorce and separation rates for TBI individuals and their partners appear to be higher than for those in the general population, as high as 78% in one study (e.g., Thomsen, 1984).

In the family support program, partners reported being distressed by the mood disturbances, the behavioral changes, and the decreased social competency that the TBI individuals displayed. They stated that it was these impairments that led to a lack of reciprocity in their relationships. For example, Derek's partner Kate was initially very positive about the future of their relationship. Over time, however, she became increasingly aware of Derek's socially inappropriate behavior. This behavior ultimately resulted in an unbalanced relationship whereby she felt as though she had another child to train. Similarly, Patrick would talk about his concerns with his partner for extended periods of time, forgetting that she had problems of her own. These sorts of problems were extremely distressing for many partners, some of whom subsequently requested assistance from the therapist to improve the quality of their relationships.

Over the follow-up period, two of the TBI individuals' partners decided to leave their relationships. These partners stated that they left the relationship because they could not adjust to the TBI individual's personality change and behavioral problems (e.g., anger outbursts). If the couple did decide to separate, support was offered to both parties until the readjustment had been made. In total, seven couples in the treatment group required relationship counseling.

The procedures involved in the relationship counseling are described below. The approach taken was based on that of behavioral marital therapy in which behavioral exchange, communication skills training, and problem-solving training are the principal intervention techniques (Jacobson & Margolin, 1979). This intervention has been found to produce enduring improvements in marital satisfaction (Hahleg & Markman, 1988).

Support for Partners

Before any structured intervention took place (e.g., communication skills training), the therapist spent time alone with the partner, allowing him or her to express how he or she was feeling. Many partners felt deeply guilty about the anger they felt against the TBI individual or about their own secret desire to end the relationship. They were aware that their partners had lost so much as a result of the accidents, and they did not want to "desert" them. Listening in a supportive, nonjudgmental manner helped the partners clarify what they felt and what the issues involved were (e.g., guilt at leaving a "helpless" person).

Behavioral Exchange

In the behavioral exchange programs that were utilized, both partners in the relationship carried out activities designed to please the other person. For instance, Grant decided to take his wife Christine for a walk in the evenings. Christine, in turn, accompanied Grant to rugby matches. The aim of such activities was to encourage "warm feelings" and a sense of collaboration between partners (Schmaling, Fruzzetti, & Jacobsen, 1989).

Communication Skills Training

Communication skills training has been described in detail elsewhere (e.g., Schmaling et al., 1989). In the family support program, communication skills were taught in order to enable the partner to clearly inform the TBI individual about the nature of the problems and describe potential solutions to these problems. The DESC system was found to be very useful for achieving this objective. DESC is an acronym for Describe the problem, Express how it makes you feel, Specify what changes are needed, and state the positive Consequences if the changes are made. In some cases, partners also needed to be taught basic assertiveness skills so that they could set appropriate boundaries about what they wanted or did not want. An example of the DESC system is given below.

Describe the problem.

Example: Peter, I have noticed that the garbage is not being put out and the dishes are not being done.

Express how it makes you feel.

Example: When I smell rotten garbage and come home to dirty dishes, I feel very angry.

Specify what changes are required.

Example: I would appreciate it greatly if the breakfast dishes could be done by lunchtime and the garbage put out each day.

Consequences.

Example: If these things were done, then the place would be cleaner and I would feel much happier when I come home.

Problem-Solving Training

In some cases, it was necessary to carry out problem-solving training. Detailed description of this procedure is beyond the scope of this chapter. An excellent description of the technique can be found in Hawton and Kirk (1989). Applied to a range of relationship problems following TBI, problem-solving procedures proved to be very effective. For example, after his accident, Derek had become restless and agitated in his sleep. As a result, Kate was not able to sleep and was quickly becoming tired and stressed. A problem-solving exercise resulted in their putting an additional single bed in their bedroom. This stratagem allowed Kate to sleep with Derek if she wished but to move to the single bed if she became too tired.

Psychosexual Counseling

None of the couples in the family support program requested formal psychosexual counseling. Psychosexual problems did occur, but it was unusual for them to be the primary cause of concern. The main intervention strategies employed for psychosexual problems were education and reassurance. For example, Susan had become more interested in sexual contact after her injury. Glen, her husband, confided to the therapist that he was frightened that this meant she would become a nymphomaniac or have an affair with another man. After he was reassured that she was unlikely to do so, the couple actually went on to establish a physical relationship more mutually satisfying than it had been prior to the accident. Unfortunately, not all sexual problems resolved this easily, and some partners reluctantly decided to limit sexual contact or cease it altogether. Other workers have also noted that partners of brain-injured men tend to dislike having intimate contact with them (Lezak, 1978, 1988; Rosenbaum & Najenson, 1976).

Intergenerational Relationships

Relationships between TBI individuals and their parents, or between TBI individuals and their children, are referred to as "intergenerational relationships."

The TBI individuals and their families reported that discord occurred in both these types of intergenerational relationships. The techniques for enhancing the relationship between TBI children and their parents and between TBI parents and their children will be discussed in turn.

TBI Children and Their Parents

Several of the participants in the study were young adults living at home with parents at the time the TBI was sustained. Parents found it hard to adapt to the sudden change in their roles that was brought about by the TBI. Just at the time offspring were reaching independence and no longer required intense parental attention, the TBI occurred and considerable parental care was again necessary. When the TBI child's functioning improved, parents then had to revert to less intensive involvement with the child. Moreover, parents now had very real fears concerning their child's ability to cope or fears concerning the possibility that a second accident would occur. As a result, some parents restricted the child by instituting a curfew (e.g., requiring him to be home by 9 P.M.) or by refusing to allow him to engage in certain activities (e.g., staying the weekend at a friend's house). These restrictions led to ongoing arguments. Richard and Aaron, for example, were furious when they were no longer allowed to be alone in their homes for a weekend while their parents were away. Arguments over driving and curfews dominated Joseph's family for many months, and Brian's mother was horrified when he announced he wanted to live independently.

In some families, the noninjured siblings resented the amount of attention the TBI child received and reacted with acting-out behavior (e.g., temper tantrums, hitting, crying). Brooks (1991) notes that it is not uncommon for noninjured siblings to be at risk of feeling jealous of the TBI child and developing behavioral disturbances. When noninjured siblings began to act out, the parents were advised to spend regular time each week with the child without the TBI child present. Family rules needed to be maintained, however, and not disregarded because parents felt sorry for the noninjured child.

Summary of the Procedure for Enhancing TBI Child–Parent Relationships

1. Reassure parents that conflict between parents and adolescents is "normal" and occurs in most families.
2. Discuss with parents the role changes that can occur for parents following TBI.
3. Encourage the parents and the TBI child to communicate clearly to each other about the problems they experience.

4. Teach parents to reappraise the TBI child's behavior (e.g., "He's trying to prove he can be independent," not "He's doing this to hurt us"). TBI children also need to be taught to reappraise their parents' behavior (e.g., "I guess they're worried about whether I'll get hurt again," not "They just don't want me to do anything").
5. Set up family conferences in which all the family meet together and engage in problem-solving exercises aimed at resolving any problems that have arisen (for a description of this procedure see Hawton & Kirk, 1989).
6. Encourage TBI children to prove to their parents that they are indeed trustworthy. This can be achieved by the TBI child regularly undertaking activities such as cooking meals, washing clothes, and getting up on time in the morning.
7. Where necessary, set up written agreements between the TBI child and the parents, outlining what acceptable rules are and what the consequences are if the rules agreed upon are not observed.

TBI Parents and Their Children

Relationships between the TBI parents and their children were also problematic at times. The problems that occurred ranged from minor difficulties such as low-level irritability toward the children to more extreme behavioral problems. Derek, for example, resented his partners' children, and at times would be verbally aggressive toward them. One of the children commented that she was cold, only to be told by Derek, "I'll put a match to you and that will warm you up." Not surprisingly, the child was frightened by this statement. When asked about the incident, Derek maintained that it was a harmless comment made to a child who whined too much and "deserved it."

In general, younger children found it hard to understand the changes in a TBI parent who still looked the same. In such circumstances, the therapist would work with the parents to generate simple explanations that their children could comprehend. One child began playing hospitals with dolls that had sore heads; another drew pictures of aliens with enlarged heads. When this happened, the noninjured partner would join them in their play and use it as an opportunity to allow the children to express their feelings and concerns. Arrangements were made for the TBI parent to spend pleasant time with each child (e.g., playing simple card games). The partner would also make sure to spend time with the children without the TBI parent present. This allowed children to receive the noninjured parent's full attention, even if only for a few brief minutes each day. It was recommended that any necessary child discipline not be carried out by the TBI parent, as experience indicated that they tended to punish severely in an inconsistent manner or give rewards noncontingently.

Summary of the Procedure for Enhancing TBI Parent–Child Relationships

1. Work closely with parents to design a method of explaining to the children what TBI is and how TBI affects their father's or mother's behavior. Possible methods of making such explanations include the use of simple verbal explanations or drawings or incorporating explanations into the children's play.
2. Ensure the safety of the children, particularly if the TBI parent's behavior is unpredictable or abusive. This aim can be achieved by the noninjured parent's remaining present when the children are with the TBI parent.
3. Encourage the children to express how they feel about the TBI parent and what has happened.
4. Arrange for the TBI parent to engage in pleasant activities with the children (e.g., going to the park, playing a game together).
5. Ensure that the children have at least a few minutes each day alone with the noninjured parent. This allows children to receive their noninjured parent's full attention, even if only briefly.
6. If the TBI parent is harsh or inconsistent in disciplining the children, encourage the noninjured parent to take responsibility for their discipline.

REDUCING DEMANDS ON FAMILY MEMBERS

Being involved in the care of an individual affected by TBI is a major responsibility (DeBoskey & Morin, 1985). Care is usually provided by the family, as the majority of TBI patients return home on discharge from the hospital (Liss & Willer, 1990). Families are often described as going through a process of mourning in which they must adjust to the loss of the person they once knew and readjust to the TBI individual's new behavior and personality (Zeigler, 1987). Families not only have to readjust to personality changes, but also are often faced with loss of income, social isolation, and the ongoing burden of dealing with the TBI individual's emotional and behavioral problems (Brooks et al., 1986; Liss & Willer, 1990; Rogers & Kreutzer, 1984). Not surprisingly, many family members eventually display signs of stress such as anxiety, depressed mood, and sleeplessness (Livingston et al., 1985a; Panting & Merry, 1972; Oddy et al., 1978a). The stress experienced by families can be reduced by decreasing the day-to-day demands they face. The following section describes the techniques utilized in the family support program to reduce demands upon families.

Accessing Resources

Community agencies and hospital outpatient clinics provide a number of services that can greatly assist families and individuals affected by TBI. Unfortunately, these services were often not accessed because families in the study had not been informed of their existence. Alternatively, the families knew that help was available but doubted whether it was worthwhile to make requests to what appeared to be an adversarial and complex system. Hence, there was a need to assist families to access existing community services. In the course of the study, participants were assisted to obtain services offered in the areas of financial assistance, vocational placement, peer support, health, transportation, and substance abuse counseling services. Information was collected on a wide variety of service-related topics such as how to access hospital files, how to obtain driving assessments, how to file insurance compensation claims, and how to obtain "fitness to drive certificates." In addition, attendant care services were arranged and monitored for some TBI clients. This monitoring was to ensure that families continued to receive services and proved critical, as there was a tendency for service agencies to underestimate the long-term impact of TBI and terminate services prematurely. Assisting families to access and maintain resources not only helped the families, but also meant that positive working relationships were established with many community agencies.

Crisis Intervention and Case Management

Many family members were concerned that they would not be able to gain assistance from health care services quickly should a crisis occur. One of the primary needs expressed by families was to know that backup assistance and support was available should it be needed. In order to provide such support, two strategies were implemented, a crisis intervention service and a case management system. The crisis intervention service offered assistance within 72 hours of a request for help. Within this time period, the therapist would make personal contact with the family involved and, after assessing the situation, arrange whatever services were necessary. In the areas within 60 miles of the university clinic, contact was usually made well within 24 hours. The crisis intervention service operated throughout the duration of the program, but was in fact utilized infrequently. Crisis intervention was most useful in cases in which a catastrophic reaction had occurred and the TBI individual had become aggressive or suicidal.

The case management system was developed in acknowledgment that the problems following TBI are long-term (Godfrey et al., 1993b) and will not resolve in 8–10 sessions of time-limited intervention. The format utilized was very similar to that documented by Intagliata, Willer, and Egri (1988). A case manager was appointed who was responsible for assessing the needs of the family and the TBI individual, assisting participants' access to services, providing assistance with problem solving, being available for crisis management, and operating as a liaison person between all the health professionals involved in the care of the TBI individual. Case managers were selected on the basis of their knowledge about TBI rehabilitation and their rapport with the TBI individual and family. For the purposes of this research protocol, the therapist was case manager for all but two of the cases.

Case managers were responsible for making follow-up visits at the very least every 12 weeks during the 2-year follow-up period and more regularly if it was deemed necessary (e.g., weekly). Visits were made to the home to ensure that contact was made with the whole family network. Experience indicated that telephone contact alone did not elicit sufficient information to gauge how the family was coping. Some family members reported over the phone that they were coping well, yet follow-up home visits clearly indicated that they were not.

During the visits, the following areas were assessed: work performance, cognitive functioning, mood disturbances, behavioral functioning, levels of social contact, and family member coping (see Appendix G). Family members' close contact with the TBI individual meant that they were frequently the first to recognize problems, identify changes in the TBI individual's needs, and notice problems that were not seen by case managers who saw the TBI individuals less frequently (for an excellent discussion of case management systems, see also Intagliata et al., 1988). The visits provided an opportunity for both the TBI individual and the family members to ask questions and express concerns they had about their present circumstances. In general, the family members and the TBI individual were seen separately so that they could discuss their concerns in private. Family meetings were arranged when specific issues needed to be addressed (e.g., how to handle the TBI individual's suicidal comments).

The follow-up visits were made regardless of whether the TBI individual and the family members reported that they were coping well or not. The fact that visits occurred regularly and not only at the request of the family constituted an effective preventative strategy for a client group in whom problems can arise unexpectedly. It also provided family members with a regular and predictable source of support. Case monitoring was found to be a highly effective means of offering ongoing support and resolving problems while they were still at a subclinical level and not yet causing any major difficulties.

Providing Emotional Support

The provision of emotional support to family members was important in helping them cope with the demands they faced. Provision of emotional support was ongoing and included a variety of strategies such as normalization, reassurance, encouraging realistic expectations, allowing emotions to be expressed, and reinforcing coping strategies. These techniques are described below.

Normalization involves providing family members with information so that they recognize that what they feel, and how they act, is similar to how other family members feel and act. The aim of normalization is to ensure that family members do not feel they are performing inadequately compared to other people in the same situation. For example, Aaron's mother had the thought that it might have been better if Aaron had been killed in the accident. This thought made her feel intensely guilty. When the therapist normalized this experience by explaining that other mothers had experienced similar thoughts, Aaron's mother immediately felt less guilty.

Reassurance involves the use of verbal statements designed to reduce fear and give hope regarding a positive outcome to a problem. For example, Annette's mother was concerned that her daughter's brain was "deteriorating" because Annette had been repeating questions. The therapist reassured her by stating that this repetition was occurring because of Annette's short-term memory deficit. As a result, the mother became less anxious.

Assisting families to form realistic expectations involves providing the family with information about the severity of the TBI member's injury and about what is appropriate to expect from him or her with respect to behavioral, vocational, emotional, social, and cognitive functioning. It also involves providing feedback to the family by informing them when they are expecting the TBI member to perform a task that he or she is not capable of performing. The aim of assisting families to form realistic expectations is to alleviate the distress families feel when the TBI member's level of functioning does not match their expectations. For example, Derek's partner Kate became extremely frustrated when he was unable to control his anger. Derek had a severe TBI with frontal lobe damage and had been out of the hospital for only 5 weeks. The therapist provided feedback to Kate about the fact that she had inadvertently expected too much from Derek, given the severity of his injury and his phase of the recovery. The therapist also spent time outlining what Kate could reasonably expect (i.e., a slow decline in the number of anger outbursts across the next 12 months). This information enabled Kate to form more realistic expectations, and her level of frustration decreased.

Providing families with the opportunity to express how they feel involves providing a setting in which family members can safely express their feelings about the TBI member's behavior and about what has happened after the TBI. The therapist simply listens empathetically and does not offer any negative comments about the TBI member's behavior or about the other family members' feelings. For example, Kate had felt angry at Derek because he no longer considered what she wanted in their relationship. However, she had not expressed this feeling because his cognitive impairment was such that he would not have understood what she said. She expressed her feeling to the therapist in private and reported feeing much better for "just having said it to someone."

Reinforcing coping strategies involves the therapist's making positive comments to the families when they had utilized an effective coping strategy. For example, Richard's parents decided that they needed to take a holiday, as they had become tired after caring for Richard in the first 4 months after his accident. The therapist verbally reinforced them for doing this.

Pragmatic Interventions

Many of the interventions that successfully reduced the demands faced by family members involved making practical changes. For instance, Susan had managed the accounts for her husband's business prior to the TBI, but following her injury she no longer had the organizational skills to do so. Her husband struggled to complete this task in addition to running his business. A simple reassignment of tasks whereby the business accounts were sent to an accountant relieved the pressure he was under. Other practical changes involved keeping the family well informed regarding health professionals' involvement, enlisting social networks to give assistance (e.g., neighbors, friends), and scheduling free time. Free time was crucial for family members if they were to be able to maintain friendships and have time to relax. Some family members arranged for weekends away while the TBI member stayed with relatives. This practice was so effective that several families followed it regularly. Support in the form of attending local head injury society meetings was advantageous, although unfortunately many rural communities did not have such a support group in the area.

Instruction in behavior management skills also helped relieve demands on family members. However, the behavior management skills needed to be implemented consistently. Derek, for instance, initially set a goal of carrying out self-care tasks (e.g., laying out his own towel for showering). His partner was instructed to compliment him whenever he completed the tasks. Unfortunately, this procedure was carried out during the week when he lived with his de facto partner, but not on weekends when he was with his parents. Teaching the procedure to his parents resulted in his self-care skills increasing and reduced the demands on his partner, whom Derek had been accusing of being "a dragon."

Coping with relatives who gave unsolicited advice was another area of stress for family members. For example, Derek's partner was repeatedly told by her mother that she should leave the relationship, while Derek's parents simultaneously told her she needed to be assertive with the health professionals who were "ripping [her] off." Simply ensuring that she spoke to family members only when she felt able to cope with the advice, and helping her to see that they were also struggling to come to terms with the TBI, helped relieve the stress she felt.

WHEN FAMILIES PRESENT BARRIERS TO EFFECTIVE REHABILITATION

There are times when families' beliefs and actions can present serious barriers to the successful reintegration of TBI individuals into the community. Families may have difficulty accepting the TBI individuals' reduced capacity and set goals and expectations based upon preinjury performance standards (Brooks, 1991). For example, Michael's partner was convinced that he would be able to return to his previous position as an engineer. Because of this belief, she discouraged Michael from attending an agricultural training program and persuaded him to begin his own business. Michael's business failed, but only after two years, during which time his finances and his self-esteem suffered considerably.

When family members are reluctant to accept the changes that have occurred following TBI, they fail to encourage the TBI member to readjust his goals (McKinlay & Hickox, 1988), they report improvements where none has occurred (Brooks, 1991), they refuse to learn the strategies they need to care for the TBI member (J. R. Johnson & Higgins, 1987), and they become reluctant to share information with health professionals, whom they view as overly pessimistic (J. R. Johnson & Higgins, 1987). As a result, the TBI member is encouraged to undertake tasks for which he does not have the skills, and failure results. The family in turn becomes frustrated and angry at what is often perceived to be the TBI member's lack of motivation and stubbornness.

The family may also take over the TBI member's responsibilities, rather than encourage independence by allowing the TBI member to complete tasks for himself. Such action is rewarded, as family members frequently complete tasks more rapidly and competently. Similarly, families may attempt to ensure the TBI member's safety (e.g., by not allowing adolescents out with friends or by controlling finances), but in doing so limit the TBI member's independence. This restriction of freedom results in the TBI member's failing to learn the consequences of his actions and remaining dependent upon the family for longer. Some of the barriers that families may present in the process of rehabilitation and the strategies utilized in the family support program to overcome these barriers are described below.

Summary of the Procedure for Overcoming Barriers to Effective Rehabilitation

1. *Family's belief:* The TBI member will recover to his preinjury level of competency.
   Family's behavior: The family members encourage the TBI member to meet preinjury goals.

Effect on TBI member: The TBI member undertakes tasks that he is not able to accomplish. The TBI member may ultimately fail and become depressed.
Alternative strategy: Utilize the guided realization technique with family members. Discuss what are realistic expectations with the family.

2. *Family's belief:* The TBI member will not be able to look after himself and will put himself at risk of harm.
Family's behavior: The family restricts the choices the TBI member can make, refuses to allow him to go out alone, or does not allow him to participate in certain activities (e.g., running). The family may also begin to focus solely on the TBI member and neglect their own social activities.
Effect on TBI member: The TBI member has a limited range of life experiences and reduced quality of life. Limited opportunity is available for the TBI member to acquire decision-making skills or to learn from the consequences of his behavior.
Alternative strategy: Work with the family to help them conceptualize their role as teachers rather than protectors. Negotiate with the family limits that offer safety but give the TBI member opportunity to learn. The TBI member can be given a series of tasks (e.g., coming home by an agreed-upon time) to prove his responsibility to family members.
3. *Family's belief:* This task needs to be completed successfully and quickly, so I had better do it myself. If I let the TBI member do it, he will be too slow and make too many mistakes.
Family's behavior: The family takes over the TBI member's responsibilities and carries out tasks for him.
Effect on TBI member: The TBI member becomes increasingly dependent upon the family. The TBI member may become angry and depressed as he feels he has no role within the family.
Alternative strategy: Ensure that the TBI member is included in family decision making. Allow the TBI member to have a number of tasks to complete, even if doing so takes additional time.

IMPLEMENTING INTERVENTIONS TO FOSTER FAMILY ADAPTATION

Families face a plethora of challenges as they attempt to adapt to the effects of TBI. The ultimate goal is for the family, in the face of all the challenges, to accept the realities of traumatic brain injury, remain responsive to the TBI family member, and keep the aspirations they hold for their own lives (Klonoff & Prigatano, 1987). To assist families to achieve this goal, the therapist had to work with tact and empathy. It was essential to establish good rapport so that family members felt able to express their feelings and request assistance when needed. Work with families proceeded at the rate determined by the families themselves, and in most cases, the initial months focused solely on laying the groundwork for future intervention (Zeigler, 1987). Later, more structured intervention was required as difficulties became apparent and of concern to families. Families were most strongly motivated for change when they themselves perceived the need, rather than when the therapist considered that there was a problem that needed addressing. It was important to ensure that families were not pressured to take on too much responsibility in the care of the TBI member. Finally, it was critical to support the family members and ensure that they had adequate resources to help them successfully meet the demands they faced.

7

Evaluation of Outcome Effects

INTRODUCTION

The family support program was developed partly in response to recommendations about the design of traumatic brain injury (TBI) services suggested in the literature. First, the literature reviewed suggests that there is a need for psychosocially oriented programs in which both the family and the TBI family member participate (Forssmann-Falck & Christian, 1989; Rosenthal, 1989). Second, in line with the promising results of Prigatano et al. (1984) and Rattok et al. (1992), rehabilitation needs to be holistic; that is, it needs to target a wide range of areas of functioning (e.g., social, family, behavioral, emotional, and cognitive), using a variety of techniques (e.g., cognitive behavioral therapy, vocational counseling, cognitive compensation). Third, contact with services needs to reflect the long-term nature of TBI sequelae (e.g., Thomsen, 1984) and thus be provided for several years after injury. Fourth, careful attention needs to be paid to the requirements of those living in rural areas where rehabilitation services are frequently either not available or difficult to access (C. Evans & Skidmore, 1989).

FAMILY-BASED REHABILITATION

The family support program involved providing ongoing comprehensive rehabilitation services to TBI victims, and their families and friends, in the home environment. The services provided have been described in detail in Chapters 3–6. An overview of these strategies is presented in Appendix C. The majority of rehabilitation strategies employed were cognitive behavioral techniques that have previously been found to be readily applicable to patients with TBI (Cicerone, 1989). The program was implemented by a graduate clinical psychology student who served as the therapist under the supervision of two senior clinical neuropsychologists with extensive experience in TBI rehabilitation. Families participating in the support program initially received four education sessions, each lasting 1 hour. They were then visited regularly during a 2-year follow-up period (mean = 21.3 months), and additional intervention was implemented for each family as needed. The average number of contact hours spent with each family was 27.6 hours (SD = 11.3), with a total of 387 contact hours being provided to the treatment group as a whole.

Although similar family-based programs have been used successfully in the management of autism (Howlin & Rutter, 1989) and schizophrenia (Falloon, Boyd, & McGill, 1984), the TBI literature tends to commend the concept of family involvement but contain very few reports of its actual use (Shaw & McMahon, 1990). The lack of family-based rehabilitation is particularly surprising given the rapid growth in number of TBI services and the fact that most TBI patients live at home during their postacute rehabilitation. The provision of support in the home environment as part of this program represents a radical difference from existing outpatient and inpatient program practices.

The major advantage of a family-based approach to rehabilitation is that support can be given to the family members with the aim of ameliorating the chronic distress they often experience (Livingston et al., 1985a,b). A further advantage is that family-based rehabilitation has the potential to prevent the regression to poorer adjustment seen in clients in rural centers who have no access to services because of economic and transportation barriers (see Prickel & McLean, 1989). Generalization of gains is also enhanced (Jacobs, 1989) by allowing TBI individuals to use their usual environment to practice new skills (Malkmus, 1989). Family-based rehabilitation enables close liaison with families and friends, which is hard to establish in inpatient and outpatient clinic settings (Sherr & Langenbahn, 1992) The costs involved in providing community-based services are considerably less than those for inpatient rehabilitation or outpatient day hospitals. In 1982, the estimated daily cost for inpatient treatment in the United States stood at $500 (Cope & Hall, 1982). While a cost–benefit analysis of family-based rehabilitation has yet to be made, there is little doubt that the financial cost is substantially less than the aforecited cost for inpatient treatment. Finally, the alienation from social networks, dependency, and deculturalization that can occur with residential programs are avoided (see C. Evans & Skidmore, 1989).

EVALUATING THE EFFICACY OF FAMILY-BASED REHABILITATION

Selecting a Research Design

Selecting an appropriate research design to evaluate rehabilitation programs for TBI individuals and their families is problematic (Baddeley, Meade, & Newcombe, 1980). For example, TBI samples are typically heterogeneous due to the diversity of brain injury (Volpe & McDowell, 1990), it is often difficult to describe a sample adequately because of a lack of (adequate) records, and, perhaps most problematic of all, ethical considerations restrict the use of random assignment to no-treatment control groups. Our study employed a nonequivalent control group design (Campbell & Stanley, 1966). A group of TBI individuals and their relatives who had participated in an earlier cross-sectional following-up study and were assessed at 6 months after injury were employed as a control group (see Godfrey et al., 1993b). The choice of this control group determined the timing of the first assessment and restricted the choice of outcome measures to those employed in the earlier study. This control group had received standard hospital care, with virtually no long-term follow-up or family-based rehabilitation. The functioning of the control group was compared to the functioning of a second group of TBI individuals and their families who were recruited during 1990 to 1991 and who participated in the family support program. Table 7.1 summarizes this design. As noted by Campbell and Stanley (1966), nonequivalent control group designs are useful when ethical constraints preclude the use of random assignment to groups (as was the case in this study). However, a possible limitation of this design is maturation–selection interaction effects that can occur, particularly if the subjects are self-selected (Campbell & Stanley, 1966). This problem can be significantly reduced if the control and treatment groups are recruited in a similar manner and matched on their pretest scores (Campbell & Stanley, 1966), as was the case in this study.

TABLE 7.1. Summary of Research Design

Control group	Family support program
Date of traumatic brain injury	
January 1988–December 1988	July 1990–September 1991
First assessment	
6 months postinjury	6 months postinjury
Intervention	
Standard hospital care	Family support program
Second assessment	
2 years postinjury	2 years postinjury

Recruitment

TBI Individuals

During the period from January 1985 to December 1988, a controlled cross-sectional outcome study was carried out with 66 TBI patients who had been admitted to Dunedin Public Hospital, Dunedin, New Zealand, and had subsequently been discharged in a conscious state (Godfrey et al., 1993b). Of these 66 individuals, 24 had been injured during 1988 and had either been admitted to the Dunedin Public Hospital Neurosurgical Unit or been seen by a unit neurosurgeon at other hospitals in the area (e.g., Kew Hospital, Invercargill). These hospitals are located in rural areas, and each has a catchment area of approximately 130,000. After being invited by letter to participate in a follow-up study, these 24 individuals had been assessed approximately 6 months after injury. They and their relatives were recontacted by letter during 1990 and asked to participate in a second follow-up assessment. Informed consent was gained from 20 individuals, who were then assessed at approximately 2 years after injury. They formed a control group subject pool and were matched on a case-by-case basis with family support group subjects (see Appendix D for details of the case-by-case matching).

A total of 14 family support group subjects were recruited from Dunedin and Invercargill Public Hospitals during the 15 months from July 1990 to September 1991. TBI individuals and their relatives were either approached immediately prior to discharge or contacted by letter soon after discharge. Family support program aims and requirements were fully explained, and a written handout describing the study and program was provided. TBI individuals and relatives were given the option of participating, declining to participate, or delaying their decision for approximately 8 weeks. If they decided to delay their decision, the family was contacted again by telephone after the 8-week period. Informed consent was obtained from all those who agreed to participate. All participants were advised that they could withdraw from the family support program at any point.

TBI individuals were selected if they were between the ages of 15 and 40, conscious on discharge from the hospital, able to communicate verbally, and had no premorbid history of psychiatric disorder, neurological disorder, or previous moderate or severe head injury. Injury severity was determined using duration of posttraumatic amnesia (PTA) and the Glasgow Coma Scale (GCS) on admission (Jennett & Teasdale, 1981; W. R. Russell, 1932, 1971). It has been found that in some circumstances, the use of PTA is preferable to the use of GCS scores, as PTA avoids the difficulties inherent in assessing coma, such as the complicating effects of extracranial factors, alcohol levels, sedation, and intubation (Bishara et al., 1992). Both duration of PTA and GCS on admission were determined by the primary physician, who assessed the TBI individual's orientation on several occasions prior to and on discharge from the hospital. TBI individuals were selected if they had sustained moderate to severe injuries, defined as a duration of PTA of greater than 1 day, or a GCS score of 9–12 (i.e., moderate injury) or 3–8 (i.e., severe injury) (Prigatano, 1992), or both.

Relatives

All TBI individuals were asked to nominate a "relative" who was willing to participate in the follow-up assessment with them. A "relative" was defined as someone who knew the TBI individual well and either resided with him or had had contact with him at least once during the month prior to his assessment (Partridge, 1991, p. 65). At their original 6-month assessment, 86% of the TBI individuals were accompanied by a relative. The majority of relatives were family members (i.e., parents, spouses, siblings), others being partners or friends. All relatives knew the TBI individual prior to the accident.

Nonparticipation

Four of the TBI individuals who met the criteria for inclusion in the control group declined to participate. There were no significant differences between the participating and nonparticipating individuals in terms of age, gender, marital status, GCS score on admission, neurosurgical intervention, or documented frontal damage. However, nonparticipators had significantly shorter duration of PTA ($t = -4.52$, $p < 0.001$). Clinical observation of these individuals suggested that they considered their head injuries to be inconsequential and therefore perceived no potential benefits from involvement in the program.

Sample Description

Descriptive demographic, injury, and neuropsychological variables are presented in Tables 7.2–7.4. The majority of injuries were due to traffic-related accidents (i.e., motor vehicles, motorbikes, bicycles, pedestrians). Other causes of injury were falls, sporting accidents, and assaults. Using GCS scores as criteria for injury severity (e.g., Prigatano, 1992), approximately equal numbers of individuals were classified as mildly, moderately, and severely injured (see Table 7.2). Abnormalities were detected in over half the TBI individuals for whom computerized tomography (CT) was performed, of whom approximately one quarter had some form of documented frontal lobe damage (i.e., contusion or hematoma). Neurosurgical intervention for evacuation of hematoma or surgical decompression was required infrequently. In comparison with other research (e.g., Brooks et al., 1987b), the TBI individuals were less seriously injured. However, this sample is representative of New Zealand admissions for severe TBI (Bishara et al., 1992). The Bishara et al. (1992) study also revealed that a significant subgroup of

TABLE 7.2. Injury Variables

Measure	Control group (N = 14) Mean	SD	Family support program (N = 14) Mean	SD
PTA (days)	13.4[a]	9.1	15.4	10.6
GCS score[b]				
3–8	36%	—	31%	—
9–12	29%	—	46%	—
13–14	35%	—	23%	—
Hospital stay (days)	36.4	28.4	28.1	19.9
Neurosurgery	21%	—	14%	—
CT abnormality[b]	69%	—	56%	—
Frontal damage	29%	—	21%	—
Skull fracture	57%	—	36%	—

[a]N = 12.
[b]N = 13.

noncomatose TBI individuals exist who have significant residual problems, including personality change and poor emotional adjustment (Godfrey et al., 1993b). This group has received little attention to date.

The majority of TBI individuals were young adult males, none over 45 years of age. On average, the individuals had received 4 years of high school education and were of predominantly lower socioeconomic status (see Table 7.3). Few participants were married, and approximately one third were unemployed.

The TBI individuals' estimated level of premorbid intellectual functioning on the *National Adult Reading Test* (NART) (Nelson & O'Connell, 1978; Nelson, 1982) and their level of neuropsychological functioning was assessed at 6 months after injury. This assessment included the following measures: the Mini Mental State exam (Folstein, Folstein, & McHugh, 1975), the Rey Auditory Verbal Learning Test (Rey, 1964), the Controlled Oral Word Association Test (Form A) (Benton & Hamsher, 1978), and the Paced Auditory Serial-Addition Task (Gronwall, 1977) (see Table 7.4). None of the TBI individuals showed signs of significant gross cognitive impairment on mental status examination. On average, their estimated premorbid intelligence was within the average range. Of note is the variability in the sample's level of cognitive impairment. On average, the TBI individuals evidenced a relatively mild degree of cognitive impairment. However, the large "within group" variability is consistent with the fact that a subgroup of TBI individuals evidenced moderate to severe cognitive impairment (see case descriptive information in Appendix D).

TABLE 7.3. Demographic Variables

	Control group (N = 14)		Family support program (N = 14)	
Measure	Mean	SD	Mean	SD
Age	24.5	7.9	26.1	7.1
Gender (% male)	86%	—	86%	—
Socioeconomic status				
Higher	7%	—	14%	—
Lower	64%	—	50%	—
Unwaged	29%	—	36%	—
Education (years)	11.7	1.9	11.5	1.0
Single marital status	79%	—	71%	—
Time postinjury (months)				
First assessment	6.6	0.9	6.4	0.8
Second assessment	21.5	3.5	21.3	3.6

Matching

Family support group TBI individuals were matched on a case-by-case basis with subjects from the control group subject pool. Individuals in the two groups were initially matched on injury severity variables and subsequently on the basis of demographic variables and level of neuropsychological functioning. As can be seen in Tables 7.2–7.4, very close matching was achieved on all variables, with statistical analysis (independent *t*-tests, χ^2 tests) showing no significant differ-

TABLE 7.4. Neuropsychological Variables

	Control group (N = 14)		Family support program (N = 14)	
Measure[a]	Mean[b]	SD	Mean	SD
MMS	27.7	2.5	28.4	1.5
NART	102.7	12.5	103.6	8.6
RAVLT	56.5	17.7	56.6	12.4
COWAT	37.5	12.5	35.1	12.4
PASAT	33.8	18.9	30.9	12.3

[a]MMS = Mini Mental State; NART = National Adult Reading Test; RALVT = Rey Auditory Verbal Learning Test; COWAT = Controlled Oral Word Association Test; PASAT = Paced Auditory Serial-Addition Task.
[b]N = 13.

ences between the groups on any of the variables. The high degree of similarity of the groups minimizes the chance of regression effects and selection–maturation effects associated with the use of a nonequivalent control group design (Campbell & Stanley, 1966).

Services Received

Table 7.5 details the percentage of the family support and control groups who consulted health professionals during the course of the study and the average number of contacts they made. Control group TBI individuals received very few follow-up services after discharge from the hospital. Within 2 years of injury, the only service most individuals (67%) continued to receive was irregular outpatient visits to a family physician or a consultant neurosurgeon. Two subjects did receive counseling from psychologists. One had seen a psychologist for 10 sessions approximately 10 months prior to the 2-year assessment. The other was continuing to receive irregular appointments at the time of the 2-year assessment. Of the sample, 20% also reported a single session with a vocational counselor, social worker, physiotherapist, or psychologist. No TBI individuals received any home-based rehabilitation, residential or day program treatment, or long-term outpatient rehabilitation (i.e., more than 8 months after discharge from hospital). Relatives

Table 7.5. Rehabilitation Services Received by Control Group TBI Individuals ($N = 14$)

	Appointments		
Health professional	Mean[a]	SD	%[b]
Neurosurgeon	2.4	1.4	100
Physician	3.1	4.1	80
Physiotherapist	48.2[c]	100.8	70
Occupational therapist	21.8[c]	34.9	50
Vocational counselor	3.6	5.9	50
Speech therapist	2.6	6.6	31
Neuropsychologist	3.2	4.8	29
Psychologist	25.0[d]	21.2	14
District nurse	2.3	8.3	7
Social worker	0.8	2.8	7

[a]$N = 13$.
[b]Percentage of individuals who received at least one appointment.
[c]The mean values are high because three individuals attended twice-daily appointments over a 2-month period.
[d]Two TBI individuals consulted a psychologist on a regular basis. One consulted a clinical psychologist for 10 sessions; the other consulted a school psychologist on a very frequent basis.

also received very few services; only 64% reported seeing a neurosurgeon, and 73% reported having no contact whatsoever with either psychologists or social workers. The main source of professional support for relatives was general practitioners. Of the relatives, 50% visited their general practitioner to discuss TBI-related problems during the follow-up period.

Assessment Procedure

Members of the control and family support groups and their relatives were assessed at approximately 6 months and 2 years after injury. The dates of the family support group assessments were predetermined on the basis of the time after injury at which their matched controls had been assessed. This matching procedure countered any potential interaction between severity of injury and length of follow-up. It also ensured independently timed assessments of functioning, preventing the possibility of experimenter bias in the scheduling of assessments when the support group TBI individuals were functioning more highly. The mean length of time since injury was nearly identical for both groups at both assessments. There were no significant differences between groups with respect to length of follow-up. The setting of the assessments varied. The majority of the assessments were held in the individual's home, with a minority of subjects choosing to be assessed at the Otago University Clinical Psychology Research and Training Center. All assessments were carried out by one of three trainee clinical psychologists who had no prior contact with the subjects and had not been involved in the family support program. Assessors received intensive training in the administration of the assessment measures. This training was provided by the therapist involved in the program and one of the supervisory clinical neuropsychologists. Training involved instruction in how to manage potential assessment issues, such as explaining difficult questionnaire wording to participants, and how to answer questions the participants had about the measures. As part of training, assessors role played strategies for dealing with possible difficulties that could arise during assessment (e.g., what they would do if a parent insisted on helping a TBI individual complete his questionnaire). Written instructions detailing the protocol for the assessment were provided to each assessor. During the assessments, interviewers provided whatever assistance was necessary, such as reading questionnaire items aloud and explaining word meanings. This assistance was necessary, as many participants in both groups had low levels of literacy. Assessments took approximately 3 hours, with a break being taken midway through the assessment.

Outcome Measures

The assessment of outcome following TBI is a complex task. At present, there is a lack of functionally relevant outcome measures (Gordon & Hibbard,

1992) that are sensitive to change and validly predict ability to cope (Baddeley et al., 1980). Functional rating scales and scales measuring activities of daily living have been employed, but these scales have several disadvantages. Not only are the distinctions within the scales coarse (e.g., "Can make bed without assistance" vs. "Cannot make a bed"), but many TBI individuals are able to perform the required tasks (e.g., dressing self, combing hair) even when they have sustained severe cognitive impairment (Baddeley et al., 1980). The use of neuropsychological tests as outcome measures (e.g., Wechsler Adult Intelligence Scale—Revised) has also been criticized due to the insensitivity of neuropsychological tests to change and their lack of relationship to everyday functioning (e.g., Cripe, 1989). Currently, there is increasing acknowledgment of the need to assess emotional functioning as a central aspect of long-term adjustment (e.g., Cripe, 1989).

The primary aim of the family support program was to minimize emotional dysfunction experienced by TBI individuals and their families. Consequently, this study employed scales assessing affective state and symptom-related distress. Because of the use of a historical control, the choice of measures at both the 6-month and 2-year assessments was restricted to those measures that had been used in the earlier cross-sectional follow-up study from which control TBI individuals were recruited. The outcome measures used are described below.

TBI-Symptom-Related Distress

The Symptom Distress Scale, a revised version of the Head Injury Behavior Scale (Godfrey et al., 1993b; Partridge, 1991), provided a measure of the distress due to symptoms commonly associated with traumatic brain injury. The scale contains 24 items describing problematic symptoms (e.g., impulsivity, lack of motivation, irritability) that were first rated as present or absent. In completing the scale, the TBI individuals and relatives were given assistance as necessary, in order to clarify the meaning of each item. If the problematic symptom was considered to be present, a rating of the amount of distress caused by the problem was made by using a 5-point Likert scale. The total score was calculated by summing the Likert ratings for each of the 24 items (range 0–120). Internal consistency on this scale has been found to be high. The scale is known to discriminate between TBI individuals and orthopedic controls, and it is sensitive to changes in symptom-related distress over time (Godfrey et al., 1993b). The most recent revised version of this scale is included as Appendix E.

Emotional Adjustment

The Zung Self-Rating Depression Scale (Zung, 1965) provided a measure of depressive symptomatology. In this scale, 20 items assess the affective, physiological, and psychological concomitants of depression. Respondents indicated on a 4-point scale how true each item was for them. The score for each item was added to give a total score (range 20–80). The scale has been found to be highly reliable in the New Zealand context (Knight, Waal-Manning, & Spears, 1983).

The Rosenberg Self-Esteem Inventory (Rosenberg, 1965) was administered as a measure of self-esteem. Ratings are made on 10 items of agreement concerning statements about self-worth (e.g., "I take a positive attitude to myself"). The total possible score on this inventory is 40. Previous research has shown that this measure is sensitive to changes in the self-esteem of TBI individuals over time (Godfrey et al., 1993b).

Physician Consultations

An independent measure of health care service utilization was provided by monitoring the number of visits made to a family physician (Christensen et al., 1992). At the time of the 2-year assessment, all respondents noted how many visits had been made to a family physician in response to TBI-related difficulties. The inclusion of this measure was important as an independent assessment of outcome that is less susceptible to demand effects than are self-report measures.

Awareness of Deficit

The Symptom Recognition Scale is a subscale of the Symptom Distress Scale, being the total number of symptoms the TBI individuals recognize as being problematic for them (range 0–24). Internal consistency on this scale has been found to be high, it is known to discriminate between TBI individuals and orthopedic controls, and it is sensitive to changes in symptom recognition over time (Godfrey et al., 1993b; Partridge, 1991).

OUTCOME EFFECTS FOR RELATIVES

A primary objective of the program was to prevent the family distress and burden that are so commonly associated with TBI. Thus, initially, the outcome data for relatives were examined. Relatives' distress about the TBI individuals' symptoms was assessed, as were two more general measures of emotional adjustment assessing level of depressive symptomatology and self-esteem. As an independent check on the external validity of these outcome measures, the number of visits relatives made to their physicians was also assessed. Means and standard deviations for these measures are presented in Table 7.6, and the data are presented graphically in Figure 7.1. All comparisons between groups were made using one-tailed t-tests.

A substantial effect is apparent for the symptom distress measures. Relatives

Table 7.6. Means and Standard Deviations for Relatives' Scores on the Outcome Measures[a]

	Time of assessment			
	6 months		2 years	
Measures	Mean	SD	Mean	SD
Symptom distress				
Control	12.5	13.4	19.7	17.6
Family support	12.1	14.8	10.7	15.0
Depression				
Control	34.2	6.4	32.4	5.6
Family support	31.9	6.0	28.9	5.4
Self-esteem				
Control	32.3	4.3	32.8	3.9
Family support	34.3	3.7	36.3	3.0
Physician visits				
Control	—	—	4.1	6.3
Family support	—	—	0.07	0.3

[a]Complete data were available for 12 control relatives, with the exception of number of physician visits, for which complete data were available for 10.

in the control condition evidenced an increase in symptom distress from the 6-month to the 2-year assessments ($t[24] = 2.3$, $p < 0.02$). In contrast to this worsening distress about symptoms evidenced by the control relatives, the family support group relatives' level of distress about symptoms decreased over this time period. At the 2-year assessment, the family support group relatives reported a trend toward lower levels of distress about symptoms compared with the control group relatives ($t[24] = 1.4$, $p = 0.09$). Consistent with the lower symptom distress reported by family support group relatives, this group also reported lower levels of depression ($t[24] = 1.6$, $p = 0.06$), higher levels of self-esteem ($t[24] = 2.63$, $p < 0.008$), and fewer physician visits ($t[22] = 2.43$, $p < 0.02$) at the 2-year assessment than did control group relatives.

OUTCOME EFFECTS FOR INDIVIDUALS WITH TRAUMATIC BRAIN INJURY

An important objective of the program was to improve the insight of the TBI individuals about their symptoms. Many authors have noted the difficulties of engaging clients who suffer from a posttraumatic insight disorder (Godfrey et al., 1993b), with whom it is difficult to establish realistic rehabilitation goals. Unfortunately, the gaining of insight is often associated with the onset of dysfunctional

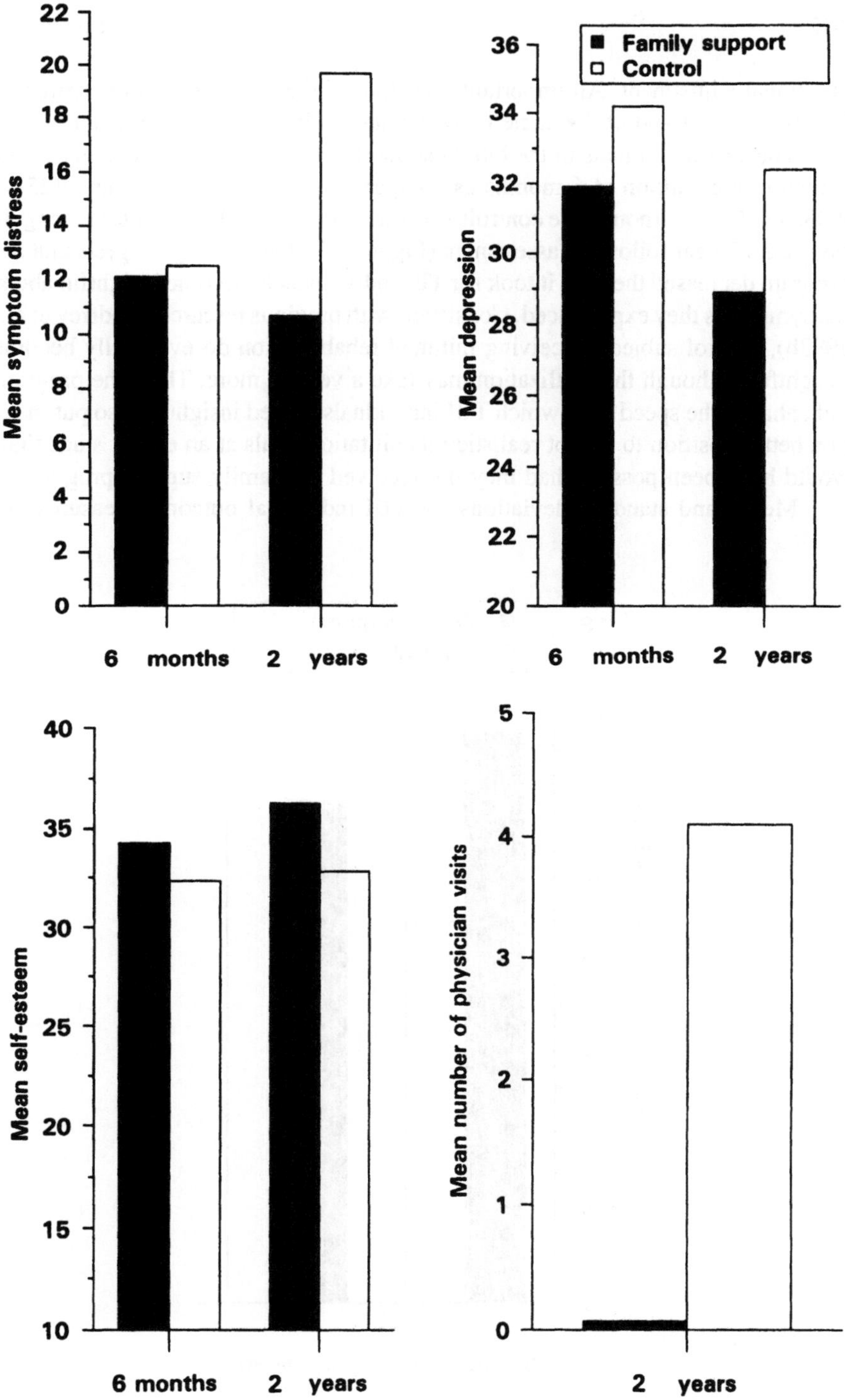

FIGURE 7.1. Relatives' mean scores on outcome measures.

emotional adjustment. An important objective of the program was to attempt to improve insight and at the same time minimize adverse emotional reactions.

The TBI individuals in the family support group showed significantly better symptom recognition at 6 months as compared with the control group ($t[25] = 2.03, p < 0.03$), although the controls showed a similar level of symptom recognition at the 2-year follow-up assessment (Figure 7.2). This finding suggests that the program decreased the time it took for TBI individuals to become insightful about the symptoms they experienced. Consistent with previous research (Godfrey et al., 1993b), control subjects receiving minimal rehabilitation do eventually become insightful, although this realization may take a year or more. Thus, the program did enhance the speed with which TBI individuals gained insight and so put them in a better position to accept realistic rehabilitation goals at an earlier stage than would have been possible had they not received the family support program.

Means and standard deviations for TBI individual outcome measures are

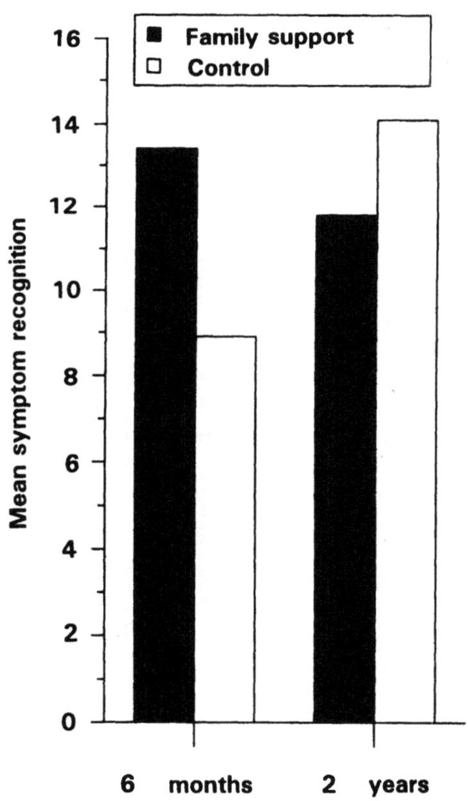

FIGURE 7.2. Mean number of symptoms recognized by TBI individuals.

presented in Table 7.7 and graphically in Figure 7.3. TBI individuals in the family support group also evidenced higher levels of depression on the Zung Self-Rating Depression Scale at the 6-month assessment ($t[25] = 1.58, p = 0.06$). Furthermore, the correlation between the family support group TBI individuals' symptom recognition scores and depression scores at 6 months was highly significant ($r = 0.82, p < 0.01$). This finding suggests that gaining of insight is associated with increased emotional dysfunction. It would seem that even with the family rehabilitation program in place, the realization that one has significant neuropsychological symptoms is inevitably associated with an increase in emotional dysfunction. The groups did not differ significantly in level of self-esteem or the frequency with which they sought assistance from their physicians.

CONSUMER SATISFACTION

Recently, greater emphasis has been placed on determining whether consumers perceive services to be acceptable and effective (e.g., Webster-Stratton, 1989). Such evaluations allow consumers of services to have an influence on the type of services they receive. The assessment of consumer satisfaction was

Table 7.7. Means and Standard Deviations for TBI Individuals' Scores on the Outcome Measures

	Time of assessment			
	6 months		2 years	
	Mean	SD	Mean	SD
Symptom recognition				
Control	8.9[a]	5.8	14.1	6.6
Family support	13.4	5.6	11.8	3.4
Symptom distress				
Control	14.6[a]	24.4	20.2	23.7
Family support	17.0	22.0	12.3	10.8
Depression				
Control	35.8[a]	7.7	38.9	10.0
Family support	40.4	7.4	39.2	8.3
Self-esteem				
Control	30.8[a]	5.0	30.3	5.8
Family support	29.3	5.2	29.6	6.8
Physician visits				
Control	—	—	3.1[b]	4.1
Family support	—	—	3.6	6.3

[a] $N = 13$.
[b] $N = 12$.

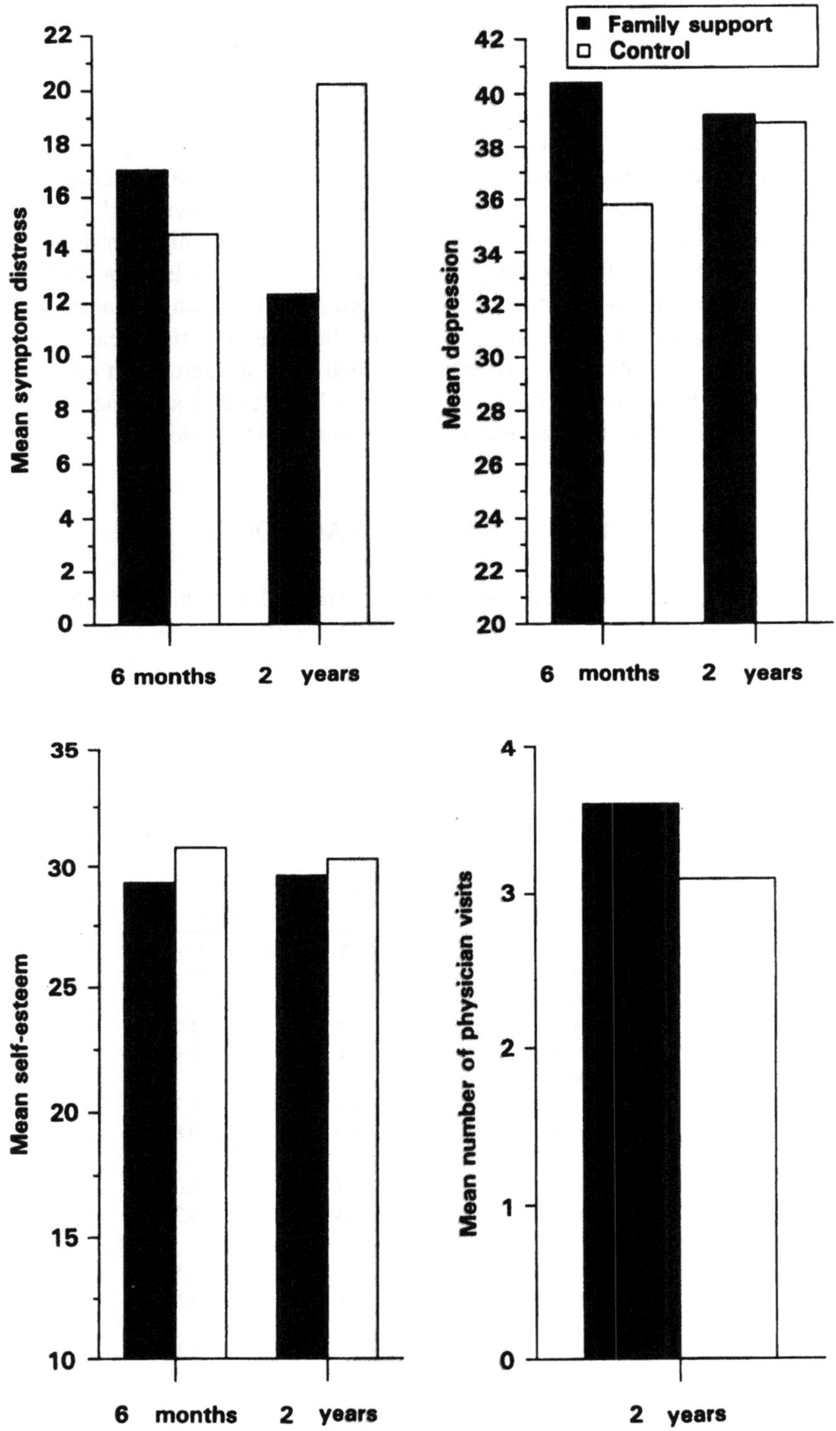

FIGURE 7.3. TBI individuals' mean scores on outcome measures.

important in this study, in which the method of service delivery was novel and involved close contact with the TBI individuals and their families over long periods. This section outlines the findings of the evaluation of consumer satisfaction. In general, very little work has been published on consumer satisfaction with services following TBI. The study by McMordie, Rogers, and Barker (1991) is one of the few published on consumer satisfaction with services following TBI. In this study, 487 members of an American head injury association were surveyed, 189 of whom returned usable questionnaires. Respondents indicated that they were not satisfied with the information provided regarding the consequences of head injury, aftercare, referral sources, and prognosis. The low level of satisfaction with the provision of information is not uncommon and has been noted by other authors (e.g., Panting & Merry, 1972; Thomsen, 1974). In addition to the findings of McMordie et al. (1991), Oddy et al. (1978a) reported that 40% of the relatives in their study also expressed concern that they were not given adequate help following the accident. The majority of these relatives thought that the level of communication between medical staff and themselves was inadequate.

In our study, consumer satisfaction was measured using a questionnaire administered at the time of the final assessment. The TBI individuals in the control group rated their satisfaction with all the services offered to them on a Likert scale with a range from 1 (not at all satisfied) to 7 (very much satisfied). Control group relatives used the same scale, but made two ratings, the first being their satisfaction with all the services offered to the TBI individual and the second being their satisfaction with all the services offered to them. The same method was used with the TBI individuals and relatives in the family support group. It was hypothesized that the family support group counterparts would report greater satisfaction with services, due to their involvement in the family support program.

As can be seen from Figure 7.4, the control group TBI individuals reported moderate levels of satisfaction with the services provided to them. Control group relatives also reported moderate levels of satisfaction with the services provided to their TBI relatives. In contrast, mean ratings given by the family support group TBI individuals and relatives were high and were significantly better than those of the control group both for the TBI individuals' ratings ($t[16] = 1.9, p = 0.04$) and for the relatives' ratings ($t[13] = 2.38, p = 0.02$). The control group relatives' mean satisfaction ratings for the services provided to them were in the low to moderate range (rating 3 or 4). Again, the family support group ratings were in the high range (rating 6 or 7). This difference between groups was highly significant ($t[12] = 3.92, p = 0.001$).

In addition to rating satisfaction with all the services offered to them, the family support group also evaluated the family support program. As can be seen in Figure 7.5, satisfaction with the family support program was very high. Participants also answered questions about their perceptions of involvement in the service, the method of service delivery, and the education component. These results are given in Appendix F.

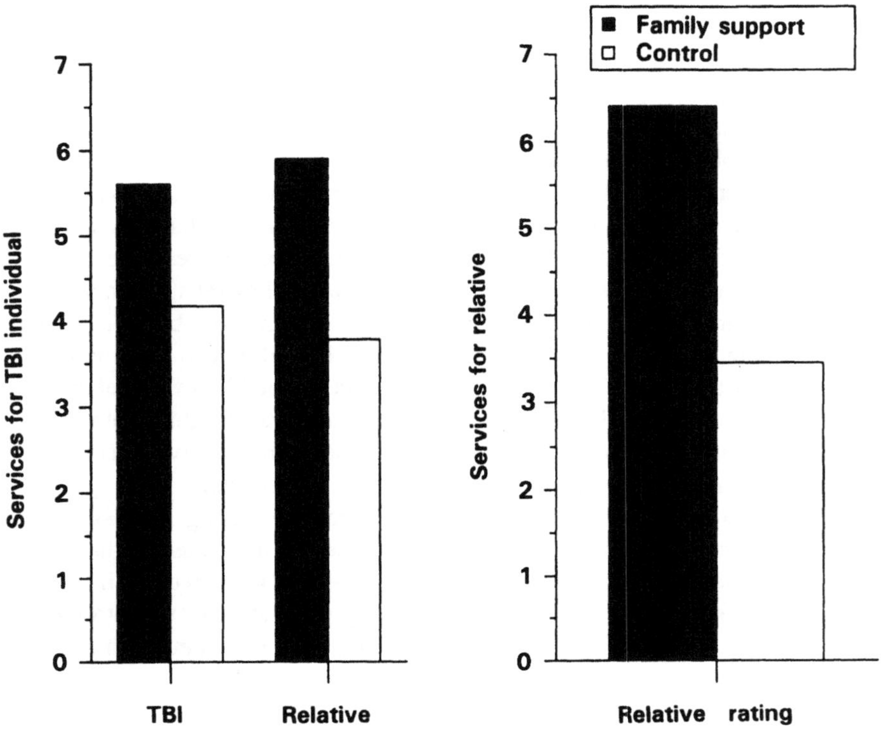

FIGURE 7.4. Mean consumer satisfaction with all services provided.

There is little doubt that family support group members perceived definite benefits from their involvement in the program. High ratings were given by both the TBI individuals and the relatives regarding the helpfulness of the advice offered. The relatives also endorsed options that indicated that involvement in the program had greatly helped both them and the TBI individual to readjust to life after head injury. The TBI individuals themselves perceived fewer benefits in terms of their adjustment, but nonetheless the majority still gave highly positive ratings. The results regarding the method of service delivery were consistent. Participants indicated a strong preference for home-based services that were available across extended periods of time. The only criticism regarding service delivery was from individuals and families who felt that follow-up needed to be available for even longer durations. In general, participants felt that they had been understood and that they had received adequate support.

Lack of information about TBI is a common concern for TBI individuals and their families. Responses to questions about information provision within the program indicate that approximately three quarters of participants were very

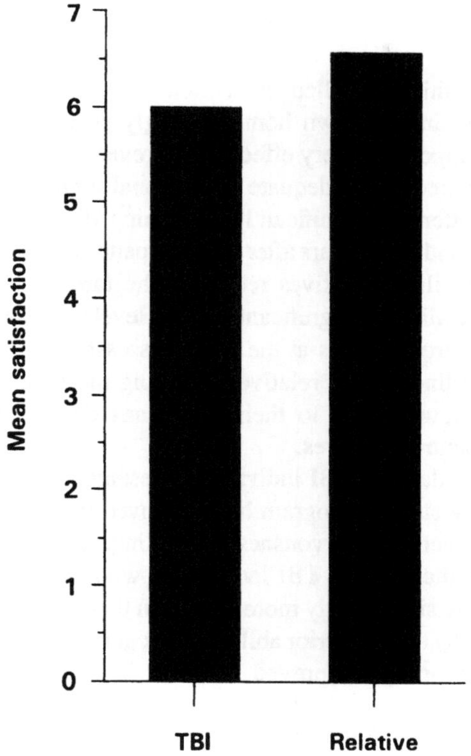

FIGURE 7.5. Mean consumer satisfaction with the family support program.

satisfied with the education provided. While education was not always easy to follow, particularly for the TBI individual, having a therapist present to discuss the information was beneficial.

Overall, the results of the evaluation of consumer satisfaction were very positive. The family support group was significantly more satisfied than the control group with services in general, and was also highly satisfied with the family support program itself. The method of service delivery (i.e., family-based with 2-year follow-up) was viewed as being very beneficial, and involvement in the program was seen to be useful in helping both the TBI individuals and their relatives cope with TBI. Interestingly, half of TBI individuals and their relatives reported that they had received more than adequate education, which for 50% of participants had greatly helped them to cope with difficulties related to head injury.

SUMMARY

The results of this controlled evaluation of the family support program provided to families in their own homes strongly support the efficacy of this approach. Family support was very effective in preventing the family burden that typifies families who receive inadequate professional support. Thus, control families evidenced a pattern of significantly worsening distress about head injury symptoms from 6 months to 2 years after injury, a pattern that was not apparent for support program families. Relatives receiving the family support program reported less emotional distress, significantly lower levels of depression, and higher self-esteem than control families at the 2-year assessment. These benefits were corroborated by the finding that relatives receiving the family support program made significantly fewer visits to their physicians during the 2 years of the program than did control relatives.

The single-case data for TBI individuals presented in earlier chapters indicated that the family support program had improved targeted problems such as low levels of social activity, nervousness, gambling, and recurrent suicidal ideation. Group data indicated that TBI individuals who participated in the family support program were significantly more insightful than controls at 6 months after injury, as evidenced by their superior ability to recognize their neuropsychological symptoms. Thus, the program proved effective in ameliorating posttraumatic insight disorder (Godfrey et al., 1993b) by decreasing the time it took TBI individuals to gain insight. A major therapeutic advantage of this "early" insight is that TBI individuals are in a better position to accept realistic rehabilitation goals at an earlier stage.

The family support program includes a number of significant advances over existing rehabilitation approaches. Perhaps the most significant of these advances is the primary emphasis on psychosocial problems rather than on improving TBI individuals' cognitive functioning. The program is designed for the entire family in recognition that family burden is a common and problematic consequence of TBI. Furthermore, the program is provided in the family home, a format that has numerous advantages including enhanced generalization of outcome effects. Finally, the emphasis on family education provides a means of improving TBI individuals' insight in a nonthreatening context. The very positive outcome data strongly support a move in service emphasis to family-based rehabilitation within a psychosocial model as the preferred method of facilitating family adjustment following TBI.

8

Summary and Conclusions

INTRODUCTION

The results of this study provide empirical support for a radical change in the type of services provided for individuals affected by TBI. First, it is suggested that rehabilitation services emphasize adjustment in the domains of social and emotional functioning, as these are the areas of functioning that prove most problematic for individuals affected by TBI (e.g., Brooks & McKinlay, 1983; Lezak, 1978). Second, it is recommended that services be provided within the context of the family system, in recognition that TBI-related problems affect the entire family (Brooks, 1984, 1991; Lezak, 1988). Third, rehabilitation should be based on a broadly conceived neuropsychosocial model (Knight, 1992) and involve the application of a *psychological intervention process* to TBI problems (Kafner & Grimm, 1980). This process involves core components of education and case monitoring, in addition to individually tailored cognitive behavioral interventions based on a functional assessment of the circumstances of the TBI individual and his family.

Our realization of the need for changes in rehabilitation emphasis came about gradually over the last decade in response to clinical and research experience at the University of Otago. Our first intervention study involved a controlled evaluation of a cognitive retraining program (Godfrey & Knight, 1985). In this study, an 8-week program of intensive memory retraining was compared with an attention-control condition. Although the memory-retraining program produced measurable improvements on memory tasks similar to those used in training, the degree of generalization to other memory tasks and to memory-related behavior in the ward environment was minimal. It was concluded on the basis of these and similar findings by other researchers that memory retraining of this sort does not produce clinically meaningful gains (Godfrey & Knight, 1987).

In contrast, our early clinical experience in attempting to rehabilitate institutionalized TBI individuals to community settings using traditional behavioral assessment and therapy approaches was proving effective (Godfrey & Knight, 1988). In the course of this clinical work, it became increasingly obvious that the adverse personality changes and emotional problems of the TBI individuals combined with the very pessimistic rehabilitation expectations of service providers represented the main barriers to the integration of TBI individuals into the community. At this time, research findings were also highlighting the significance of adverse personality change and emotional problems following TBI (McKinlay et al., 1981; Oddy & Humphrey, 1980; Tyerman & Humphrey, 1984).

Subsequent research efforts at the University of Otago attempted to define the behavioral basis and impact of personality change following TBI. Using direct observation methodology, subtle changes in verbal and nonverbal behaviors were identified that rendered the TBI individuals less rewarding to interact with (Godfrey et al., 1989). TBI individuals were judged to be particularly unskilled during the first few minutes of a novel social interaction, the very time when the other party is likely to decide whether or not to continue a conversation (Spence et al., 1993). These findings suggested that failure to reward others socially is one possible mechanism through which TBI individuals become socially isolated. Although subtle, these changes in social behavior were also found to have a significant impact on the TBI individuals' families. For example, it was found that family members had to prompt responses from socially unskilled TBI individuals during a problem-solving discussion at twice the rate of the more socially skilled controls. This finding is consistent with the notion that daily interactions with a TBI individual are likely to be exacting for family members and may represent a chronic source of stress (Godfrey et al., 1991). Taken together, these microanalytical studies of social interaction following TBI highlighted the need to address both the TBI individual's social behavior and its impact on the family during rehabilitation.

Our more recent research on posttraumatic insight disorder has similarly had an impact on the design of the family support program. This research documented the relationship between TBI individuals' awareness of their symptoms and their level of emotional dysfunction (Godfrey et al., 1993b). It is important that the period of poor symptom awareness following TBI was found to be transient for the majority of TBI individuals, consistent with the interpretation that poor insight is largely a psychological phenomenon and hence potentially modifiable through psychological (e.g., cognitive–behavioral) interventions.

The current study utilized a nonequivalent control group design to assess the efficacy of the family support program. The program was designed to alleviate symptom-related distress and to improve the emotional adjustment of TBI individuals and their relatives. TBI individuals in the family support group were closely matched on a case-by-case basis with TBI individuals in the control group for severity of injury, demographic characteristics, and level of neuropsychological functioning. Family support program participants then received a 2-year rehabilitation program that involved education, case monitoring, and cognitive–behavioral intervention. Control group participants had previously received standard hospital care, which generally comprised short-term follow-up (i.e., for periods of less than 8 months), in most instances delivered by occupational therapists and two or three follow-up appointments with a neurosurgeon. At 6 months and 2 years after injury, TBI individuals and their relatives were assessed by a trainee clinical psychologist who had no prior contact with the families or with the research study itself. The psychologist assisted families in completing questionnaires assessing symptom recognition, symptom-related distress, emotional adjustment, and health care utilization.

EFFECTIVENESS OF THE FAMILY SUPPORT PROGRAM

Outcome Effects for Relatives

Group Outcome Measures

The results of this study replicated earlier findings that indicated that without appropriate support, family distress worsens with increasing time after injury (e.g., Brooks et al., 1986; Brooks & McKinlay, 1983; Partridge, 1991). Over the 2-year follow-up period, the relatives in the control group reported significant increases in their level of distress about the TBI individuals' symptoms. This worsening distress is not surprising, given the impact that TBI has upon the entire family (Florian et al., 1991), who face the ongoing demands of adverse personality change, often with limited information and support (Klonoff & Prigatano, 1987). In contrast to this pattern of worsening distress reported by the relatives in the control group, the average level of symptom-related distress reported by relatives in the family support group remained low at the 2-year follow-up assessment. This finding is extremely encouraging in that it suggests that involvement in the family support program effectively *prevented* a family's becoming distressed about TBI symptoms.

In addition to not experiencing the usual pattern of worsening family distress about TBI symptoms, the relatives in the family support group reported better emotional adjustment than control group relatives. Thus, the self-esteem scores for the family support group relatives were significantly higher at the 2-year assessment than those reported by control group relatives. Similarly, the depression scores for the family support group were lower at the 2-year assessment compared with those of the control group relatives (this difference being only marginally significant, $p = 0.06$). These findings demonstrate that the emotional well-being of family members can be maintained, even in the face of the ongoing stress of close involvement with a TBI individual, if appropriate support is provided. Finally, the relatives in the family support group also reported having significantly fewer consultations with their family physicians regarding TBI-related concerns compared with relatives in the control group. This finding considerably strengthens confidence in the results of the self-report outcome measures. As an outcome measure, the number of family physician consultations is less susceptible to demand effects than self-report measures and thus provides an independent measure of the relatives' adjustment.

Consumer Satisfaction

The family support group relatives reported very high levels of consumer satisfaction. They were significantly more satisfied with the services offered both to them and to the TBI individual than their control group counterparts. Relatives in the family support group preferred home-based support over hospital-based support. They rated the 2-year program duration to be highly desirable. They also reported that the program had greatly helped them deal with the TBI. The education module was perceived as being easy to follow, and the presence of a psychologist who could discuss the information with them was seen as beneficial. Many relatives wrote additional comments on their forms stating how helpful they found the program and expressing the opinion that the program should be offered to other families affected by TBI. The following quotations are a selection of the many positive comments recorded on the consumer satisfaction questionnaire completed by relatives in the family support group:

> I can't imagine how difficult life would have been if [TBI individual's name] had not been a participant in this study. [Therapist's name] understanding of head injury and skill in relating to [TBI individual's name] and myself was excellent.

> We really can't say enough good things about your service . . . without this help we may have made more mistakes.

> They do a good job all around . . . they are the only service that comes to you, you do not have to approach them first.

Outcome Effects for Individuals with Traumatic Brain Injury

Single-Case Studies

The single-case data indicated that the cognitive behavioral interventions (e.g., goal setting, cognitive restructuring) were an effective means of ameliorating a range of TBI-related problems. When cognitive–behavioral interventions were applied to problems such as social withdrawal, nervousness, and recurrent suicidal ideation, substantial improvements in functioning resulted. Moreover, the improvements in functioning were maintained when the TBI individuals were reassessed at follow-up intervals of 4–6 weeks. These findings are particularly encouraging in that they demonstrate that cognitive–behavioral interventions can be successfully applied in community settings. In the past, the application of behavioral interventions to TBI-related problems has been largely restricted to residential programs, in which the degree of environmental control is very high (e.g., Wood, 1987).

Group Outcome Measures

The group outcome results for the TBI individuals were less convincing. There was a trend for the symptom distress scores of TBI individuals in the family support group to decrease across time. In contrast to this finding, the symptom distress scores of TBI individuals in the control group increased across time. However, there were no significant differences between the control group and the family support group at the 2-year assessment on measures of symptom-related distress, emotional adjustment, or number of family physician consultations. There may be a number of reasons for the apparent lack of program benefits for TBI individuals as assessed by the group outcome measures.

First, methodological constraints may have precluded the possibility of finding positive results. In particular, the study had low statistical power, reflecting both the small numbers in the groups and the large within-group heterogeneity. The methodological constraints of the study are outlined in more detail in a later section of this chapter.

Second, the program itself may not have been effective in its method of delivery. The single-case data indicated improvements in functioning when the intervention was applied in an intensive focused manner, as was the case for the cognitive–behavioral interventions for specific TBI problems (e.g., social withdrawal). However, the less intensive interventions (e.g., offering support and advice) that targeted emotional adjustment were less efficacious. It may well be that the persistent and severe problems that are experienced by TBI individuals require what has been referred to as "high-power interventions" (Sanders, 1992, p. 31). Such interventions involve concentrated contact with the therapist, very structured intervention plans, and close monitoring of progress. In contrast, some of the interventions utilized in our study were lacking power in terms of structure and number of therapy contact hours. Recent findings from acute care programs have indicated that higher-intensity interventions (i.e., 5–6 hours daily for the first 4 months) result in somewhat better outcome at discharge on functional rating scales (Spivack, Spettell, Ellis, & Ross, 1992). Whether this is also the case for postacute rehabilitation remains to be determined.

Third, the content of the family support package may not have been sufficiently comprehensive. Some strategies (e.g., cognitive remediation for attention deficits) were not implemented because of a lack of resources. Furthermore, many

TBI participants in the family support program did not receive structured vocational reentry programs, nor was it possible to utilize group therapy because of the widespread geographic location of participants.

Finally, the lack of statistically significant improvement in the TBI individuals in the family support group compared with the TBI individuals in the control group may simply reflect the fact that TBI rehabilitation techniques are not potent enough to impact positively upon the wide range of severe impairments associated with TBI. There has been increasing concern that the efficacy of skills-based rehabilitation techniques for individuals with organically based impairments (e.g., schizophrenia) may be limited. For example, it now appears that some skills-based training aimed at improving interpersonal competency neither generalizes outside the training situation nor impacts on the individual's overall quality of life (Halford & Hayes, 1991). As Eames (1992) notes, the outcome studies carried out with TBI individuals over the last 20 years are disheartening, and in view of this circumstance, the greatest hope is now placed in the possibility of limiting the damage to the brain in the acute phase of medical treatment.

Awareness of Deficit

Recent research has found that posttraumatic insight disorder occurs in the period up to 1 year after injury (Godfrey et al., 1993b, p. 503). During the first few months after injury, TBI individuals tend to underreport their TBI-related symptoms. This lack of symptom awareness can greatly impede psychosocial adjustment (Prigatano, 1986), result in adherence to unrealistic goals (McGlynn, 1990), and impede the implementation of compensatory strategies (Youngjohn & Altman, 1989). Contemporary rehabilitation approaches, including the family support program, have addressed this problem by attempting to teach TBI individuals to be more aware of their deficits (Prigatano, 1987a), providing feedback (Gross et al., 1982), and giving TBI individuals a series of tasks designed to demonstrate to them what their level of ability is (Allen & Ruff, 1990; Youngjohn & Altman, 1989). The current results indicate that these techniques are indeed efficacious in improving awareness, as evidenced by significantly higher Symptom Recognition Scale scores for TBI individuals in the family support group, when assessed 6 months after injury.

Interestingly, the TBI individuals in the family support group also reported significantly higher depression scores than the control group individuals at the 6-month assessment. Furthermore, both their self-esteem scores and their depression scores were significantly correlated with their symptom recognition scores. These results lend strong support to the notion that increased awareness is causally related to worsening emotional distress (e.g., Boake et al., 1987; Fordyce et al., 1983; Godfrey et al., 1993b). However, by the 2-year assessment, the control group's symptom recognition scores had also increased, and by this time there was no significant difference between the groups in level of either symptom recognition or depression. The possibility of worsening emotional distress as a result of "therapeutically" enhancing insight has long concerned some researchers. Generally, these researchers believe that poor insight, particularly in the early phases, may serve positive functions such as maintaining hope and motivation or increasing the TBI individual's sense of control (Deaton, 1986; Moore et al., 1989). It has also been suggested, however, that poor insight reflects adherence to premorbid performance expectations that are no longer realistic (Godfrey et al., 1994). Although such unrealistic expectations may temporarily buffer TBI individuals from emotional dysfunction, they also prevent individuals from establishing a realistic life-style that is compatible with their abilities. Furthermore, recent findings suggest that the return of insight eventually occurs even without therapeutic intervention and is inevitably associated with mood disturbance (Godfrey et al., 1993b). In summary, ignorance (of symptoms) is not bliss, nor will ignorance be maintained forever.

Consumer Satisfaction

The consumer satisfaction ratings of the TBI individuals clearly indicated satisfaction with the family support program superior to that with standard hospital follow-up care. The TBI individuals were not only significantly more satisfied with the services offered to them following the injury, but also strongly supported the long-term nature of the program. The education module was also favorably received, with TBI individuals particularly liking the opportunity to discuss the material with the psychologist. Some TBI individuals found the material difficult to follow. However, it is not possible to know whether this difficulty was due to the limitations of the education module (e.g., complexity of the language) or whether it reflected the TBI individuals' cognitive impairment at the time education was provided. The high level of satisfaction with the family support program is an exciting finding, given the low levels of satisfaction with education and with referral to follow-up services found in other studies (e.g., McMordie et al., 1991). These concerns were not evident in our research; rather, TBI individuals were consistently positive about the family support program itself, the therapist, the benefits they received from their involvement, and the method of service delivery.

METHODOLOGICAL LIMITATIONS

The study incorporated a number of methodological limitations that need to be taken into account when considering the findings. The most problematic methodological issue was the low number of subjects in each condition. This problem is exacerbated by the fact that the subjects were drawn from a population that is characterized by high levels of variability in terms of symptom type and severity (Barry & Riley, 1987; Gordon & Hibbard, 1992; Volpe & McDowell, 1990). Given this heterogeneity, larger samples are necessary if intervention-outcome studies are to have sufficient statistical power to detect clinically meaningful changes. Hence, the low numbers of subjects per group and the high level of within-group variance combined to reduce the possibility of detecting clinically meaningful improvements in adjustment for the TBI individuals (Baddeley et al., 1980). The best example of this problem is seen in the scores on the Symptom Distress Scale for the control group TBI individuals at the 2-year follow-up. On this measure, the standard deviation scores for the TBI individuals in the control group are greater than the mean scale scores. In order to obtain a statistically significant reduction in distress scores using 14 subjects, TBI individuals in the family support group would have needed to reduce their symptom distress scores to near-zero levels. It is possible, therefore, that clinically meaningful changes in functioning did occur but failed to reach statistical significance.

A second problem also occurred as a result of the small numbers in each condition. With small samples, the probability of Type 2 errors is increased, particularly where there is high extraneous variation (Minium, 1970). Type 2 errors involve incorrectly accepting the null hypothesis, in this case that the family support program had no positive effect. Unfortunately, any adjustments in alpha levels made to reduce the risk of Type 1 errors (incorrectly accepting the alternative hypothesis) further increase the risk of Type 2 errors (Minium, 1970). Therefore, on balance, it was decided to reduce the risk of Type 2 errors by keeping alpha levels at 0.05. While it is possible that Type 1 errors occurred as a result of this decision, the risk was minimized by restricting the number of comparisons made. Furthermore, the consistency of results across measures mitigates against drawing erroneous conclusions as a result of Type 1 errors. That is, none of the group outcome measures for the TBI individuals in the family support group demonstrated significant benefit, whereas all but one of the outcome measures for the relatives in the family support program demonstrated statistically significant benefits. This consistent pattern of significant findings fosters confidence that the results did not reflect chance significant findings.

The study was also limited by a number of measurement issues. First, it was decided to utilize a control group that had been assessed as part of a previous research study (Partridge, 1991). It was necessary to do this because of the limited availability of TBI individuals with moderate to severe injuries in the local region. The use of a historical control group also meant that the ethical difficulties associated with random allocation to treatment and no-treatment conditions was avoided, as the family support program had not been available for control group families at the time they were assessed. However, the decision to use this control group restricted the choice of outcome measures to those that had been employed in the prior research study. Some of these measures had a relatively low level of psychometric development. The largely predetermined choice of outcome measures also meant that a number of areas of outcome were not assessed as fully as would have been desirable. For example, no measure of interpersonal competency (e.g., the ability to initiate and maintain conversations) was included. Nor were process measures other than the Symptom Recognition Scale included.

Unfortunately, no adequate assessment was made to determine whether the relatives were actively applying the strategies taught during the family support program. Because of this deficiency, it could not be determined whether or not the improvements in relative adjustment were a result of the application of coping strategies and skills taught as part of the family support program. Such internal validity issues are difficult to address (Bowers & Clum, 1988), the assessment of internal validity being complicated by the interaction of multiple influences in clinical intervention programs (Jones, Cumming, & Horowitz, 1988). Despite these limitations, it can be concluded that regardless of the therapeutic mechanism responsible for the program benefits, relatives who participated in the family support program were on average better adjusted than relatives in the control condition.

A final methodological limitation of the study is that of the use of a nonequivalent control group design. While the case-by-case matching did much to lessen the probability of regression or maturation effects, the use of a group outcome design may itself have been inappropriate. As previously mentioned, group designs are less likely to find statistically significant results when applied to the TBI population. The reason is partly that severe TBI has a relatively low incidence, making recruitment of adequate-size samples difficult. Furthermore, measurement of functioning in this group, which is characterized by heterogeneous patterns of impairment, often results in the distribution of data that do not meet parametric assumptions (Barry & Riley, 1987; Gordon & Hibbard, 1992; Wilson, 1987; Volpe & McDowell, 1990; Zahara & Cuvo, 1984). Because of these problems, many researchers have recommended the use of single-case designs. This view is supported by the fact that the single-case data for TBI individuals in the family support program showed quite convincing intervention effects, while the improvements evident on the group outcome measures were not statistically significant.

COMPARATIVE EFFECTIVENESS OF FAMILY-BASED REHABILITATION

To date, very few controlled intervention-outcome studies have been conducted in this area. Those that have been published have tended to employ neuropsychological tests as outcome measures (e.g., Prigatano et al., 1984), precluding direct comparison with our study, which employed psychosocial outcome measures. Thus, it is difficult to evaluate the relative efficacy of the family support program compared with other rehabilitation approaches. Perhaps the most comparable intervention-outcome study is that published by Rattok et al. (1992), who compared the benefits of three different intervention mixes on outcome following TBI rehabilitation. This study included ratings of the TBI individuals' functioning by relatives in 19 areas (e.g., regulation of affect, co-operation, capacity for intimacy), as well as assessment of aspects of emotional adjustment such as self-esteem and interpersonal empathy.

In contrast to this study, the TBI individuals in the Rattok et al. (1992) study were rated as having made significant improvements on group outcome measures. However, interpretation of these findings is hampered by methodological problems. First, the ratings of TBI individuals' functioning were made by the relatives shortly after the TBI individuals had been absent from home at a day program for 20 weeks. It is possible, therefore, that the positive outcome ratings were not due to the day program per se, but rather reflected other factors such as family respite. Second, a no-treatment control group was not included in the experimental design. Therefore, it is possible that the improvement may have occurred in the absence of treatment. Finally, no follow-up data were presented to indicate that the gains made were maintained after the TBI individual was discharged from the day program. No other controlled intervention-outcome research that we are aware of has included relatives in the rehabilitation and assessed the outcome. A worthy objective for future research would be to compare the benefits of family-based rehabilitation with other rehabilitation approaches.

CLINICAL IMPLICATIONS

The results of this intervention-outcome study have a number of significant implications for current rehabilitation practices for TBI individuals and other families. The most obvious implication is the need to provide families of TBI individuals with ongoing support. The literature indicates not only that families experience ongoing affective distress (Lezak, 1978; Shaw & McMahon, 1990), but also that they are faced with changes in financial status (Liss & Willer, 1990) and alterations in role functioning (Zeigler, 1987). The prevention of family distress about TBI symptoms, the maintenance of emotional adjustment, the reduced reliance on health services, and the high consumer satisfaction ratings by relatives in the family support program lend strong support to the wider implementation of family-based rehabilitation.

A clear preference for home-based rehabilitation was indicated in the responses on the consumer satisfaction questionnaire. Home-based intervention facilitated long-term contact not only with the TBI individual but also with family and friends. This breadth and duration of contact is difficult to achieve in inpatient or outpatient settings. Yet this close contact affords a strong therapeutic relationship between the therapist and the whole family, allows the therapist to assess and intervene within the context of the family system, and ensures consistency in management approaches. Other advantages of home-based intervention included less disruption to families who have often been visiting the TBI individual in hospitals for months and greater opportunity for family members to ask questions about TBI-related issues.

A preference for long-term follow-up and support was also indicated in the consumer satisfaction evaluation. Indeed, two TBI individuals were dissatisfied with the length of follow-up, stating that the program should have been available for longer. In some cases, posttraumatic epilepsy and relationship dissolutions did not occur until over 18 months after injury. At this stage, TBI individuals and their families would normally have little, if any, contact with the health care services. However, those who received the family support program were still in contact with a therapist and able to receive support quickly. Those TBI individuals who had less severe injuries (e.g., posttraumatic amnesia of less than 7 days) often did not require the extended follow-up, and for this subgroup a shorter duration of case monitoring may be more appropriate.

The findings in this study raise two issues regarding clinical intervention with TBI individuals. The first is that the techniques utilized to increase awareness (i.e., education, feedback, guided self-discovery) appeared to be successful. This finding is extremely important, as poor insight has long been a problematic issue in TBI rehabilitation (Youngjohn & Altman, 1989) and awareness of deficits is seen to be a prerequisite for effective clinical intervention (Godfrey et al., 1993b). In many cases, the origins of lack of awareness are considered to be organic (e.g., Ridley, 1989), and hence not amenable to psychological intervention. The increased awareness found in this study indicates that applying psychological techniques to ameliorate lack of insight may well be effective for many TBI individuals. Second, cognitive–behavioral techniques are effective when they are applied on a case-by-case basis to specific TBI-related problems (e.g., lack of social activity). Careful assessment and tailoring of interventions to the problems of the particular TBI individual appear to be critical for effective intervention with this population, which demonstrates such heterogeneity in the presenting problems.

Appendixes

A

What Happens after a Traumatic Brain Injury?

SESSION 1

What is a traumatic brain injury?

Traumatic brain injuries can be divided into two types, open and closed. Open traumatic brain injuries involve piercing the skull, as might happen when a person falls onto sharp rocks. Injuries of this nature leave the brain open to the environment. Closed traumatic brain injuries, on the other hand, are the result of a blow to the head or the head hitting a flat surface (e.g., the road). In these injuries, the skull is not broken open and the brain is not exposed.

What happens to the brain in traumatic brain injury?

The blow to the head tears the cells of the brain. These cells are responsible for sending messages throughout the brain and body. When they are torn in this manner, it is called "neuronal shearing" and often involves widespread damage to the brain. Such damage is sometimes very hard to find using X rays or scans. Sometimes the damage to the brain cells is made worse by the swelling of the brain. At other times, blood vessels inside the head are torn, and the escaping blood presses against the brain. Both brain swelling and blood clots cause increased pressure on the brain.

When is a traumatic brain injury classified as severe?

The severity of a traumatic brain injury is usually measured by either the Glasgow Coma Scale (GCS) or the duration of posttraumatic amnesia (PTA). We will look at each of these in turn.

1. *Glasgow Coma Scale (GCS)*: Some people who suffer a traumatic brain injury are admitted to the hospital in a coma. When a person is in a "coma," his eyes are not open, he is unable to speak, and he does not obey simple commands (e.g., "raise your hand"). When the person is in coma, his GCS is low (less than 8/15) and the traumatic brain injury is classified as severe. As the person recovers from coma, the GCS increases up to normal full consciousness (15).
2. *Duration of posttraumatic amnesia (PTA)*: PTA refers to the length of time between the traumatic brain injury and the return of continuous memory for everyday events (e.g., who visited yesterday, what was eaten for lunch). A traumatic brain injury is severe when the length of PTA is greater than a day. The relationship between duration of PTA and severity of injury is as follows:

Duration of PTA	*Severity of injury*
Less than 5 minutes	Very mild
5–60 minutes	Mild
1–24 hours	Moderate
1–7 days	Severe
1–4 weeks	Very severe
More than 4 weeks	Extremely severe

Recovery from traumatic brain injury

It is thought that most of the recovery from traumatic brain injury occurs during the first 6–12 months after the accident. Further modest recovery then continues slowly over a period of months or years. Much of this later recovery is not due to any physical repair of the brain. It is a result of the individual and his or her family and friends learning ways of coping with the changes that result from the traumatic brain injury. The length of the recovery period and how much a person recovers differ from person to person. Research has shown that younger people tend to make a better recovery, as do those with less severe injuries. Other factors that may affect recovery include how confident the person is of recovery, his level of motivation, the occupational skills he has, his willingness to learn to do things in a different way, and the support available from friends or family.

Global outcome following traumatic brain injury

Because the brain helps control the way we think, speak, behave, move, and feel, a traumatic brain injury can affect many areas of a person's life. The ways in which a traumatic brain injury affects a person's life are collectively called "outcome." Outcome following traumatic brain injury is sometimes assessed using the Glasgow Outcome Scale (GOS). The GOS describes the following four broad categories of outcome:

1. *Vegetative*: The person shows no evidence of knowing what is happening around him or her. He or she cannot talk or obey even simple commands.
2. *Severe disability*: The person is awake and alert, but needs others to help with things like dressing, getting out of bed, or moving around the house.
3. *Moderate disability*: The person is independent, but some previous activities either at work or socially are now no longer possible.
4. *Good recovery*: The person is able to go back to normal work and social activities, *although there may be some physical or psychological problems.*

Limitations of "global outcome" measures

While global outcome measures such as the GOS are useful, they tend to be too general. Many important changes that are not detected on the GOS can occur (e.g., problems with memory or tiredness). These changes may occur even when the person has made a "good recovery." Such changes are very important for both the individual and the family and friends. For this reason, it is necessary to have a more detailed look at what you can expect to happen after a traumatic brain injury. We will begin to do this in next week's session.

SESSION 2

Outcome following traumatic brain injury

Recently many researchers have been looking at the changes that happen after people suffer a traumatic brain injury. These changes may be:

1. Psychological (e.g., differences in mood and personality).
2. Cognitive (e.g., difficulty in thinking quickly or problems with remembering things).
3. Neurological (e.g., problems with walking, vision, or balance).
4. Social (e.g., changes in work performance, leisure activities, and relationships with others).

Over the next three weeks, we will look at the changes that can occur in these four areas.

Psychological Changes

1. *Changes in personality*: After a traumatic brain injury, some people notice changes in the way they act. For example, people who were energetic before the accident may find that they now have less "get up and go," or a very even-tempered person may find that he or she is now more likely to get angry. These differences are called "personality changes." The most common of these changes are:

   (a) Becoming angry more frequently.
   (b) Being impatient and irritable.
   (c) Becoming upset easily.
   (d) Having rapid mood swings (e.g., suddenly feeling very down in the dumps for no apparent reason).
   (e) Experiencing a lack of motivation (e.g., not being bothered to complete a job).
   (f) Finding it difficult to become interested in things.

Occasionally, people may find that they are more interested in sex and are more likely to do things without thinking about them first. Below is a list of personality changes that may occur after traumatic brain injury. The majority of injured individuals experience one or more of these problems.

Area of change

Anger	Getting upset easily
Anxiety	Impatience
Boredom	Irritability
Depression	Mood change
Difficulty becoming interested in things	Quarrelsome

When will these changes happen and how long will they last?

Research has shown that people who suffer a traumatic brain injury may not worry about, or even notice, the personality changes for the first few months after the accident. The reason may be that this is the time when the person is recovering well physically, and people naturally tend to concentrate on their recovery. However, at about 1 year after the traumatic brain injury, family and friends report personality changes. These changes can be very distressing, especially when they are found to be difficult to cope with. Often for people who are affected in this way by injury, the changes will persist. However, some of the difficulties may be less frequent in number, or less distressing, by the second year after the accident. It is possible to learn ways of coping with these personality changes. Such ways of coping can help lessen the distress that these changes may cause, as well as help the individual and the family and friends find new ways of dealing with personality changes.

What causes the personality changes after a traumatic brain injury?

As mentioned in Session 1, most of the things we do are controlled by the brain. This includes control over our personality and emotions. The damage to the brain caused by a blow to the head can result in changes in the person's usual manner of behaving.

2. *Changes in mood*: Changes in mood occur quite frequently after a traumatic brain injury. "Mood" simply refers to how a person feels. There are many different moods a person can experience (e.g., sad, happy, irritable). After a traumatic brain injury, people may find that they feel more worried, sad, upset, or angry. Sometimes people will also find that how they feel changes very quickly.

When will these changes happen and how long will they last?

As with the personality changes, changes in mood do not seem to be noticed until about 1 year after the accident. At 1 year, 74% of those in a New Zealand study reported that they had experienced changes in mood; most had felt anxious or depressed. Of these people, about one in four have had serious problems with their mood. Mood seems to improve by 2 years, with only about half as many people reporting difficulties. It is helpful to know that there are a wide variety of very effective techniques that can help people to change or cope with their mood. It is a good idea to seek professional help for mood problems.

What causes the changes in mood after a traumatic brain injury?

The reasons for these changes in mood are not well understood. It seems, however, that they may result from the losses that can occur as a result of a traumatic brain injury (e.g., loss of job, ill health). This idea is supported by the fact that most mood problems happen at around 1 year after injury. At this time, many people are beginning to come to terms with the long-term effects of having a traumatic brain injury (e.g., having to accept changes in what they can do). It may also be possible that mood changes are directly caused by the injury to the brain, although this seems less likely.

Some Ideas for Coping with Personality and Mood Changes

1. Recognize that there is a problem.
2. Pinpoint the behavior that is causing the problem and describe it clearly. This will help everyone involved to know exactly what is happening.
3. Try to find out when the behavior is most likely to happen (e.g., only when the person is tired or only when the person is at home?).
4. Communicate about the problem. It is necessary to let the person know what it is about his behavior that is distressing you and then tell him specifically how he might improve it. It is also important to encourage him when a change is made.
5. Change how people react to the upsetting behavior. It is very easy to "jump in" or overreact to problem behavior. Sometimes no reaction, or a calmer reaction, is a better way to deal with it. For example, anger outbursts may stop very quickly if they are ignored.

SESSION 3

Cognitive Changes

There are many different cognitive changes that can occur after a traumatic brain injury. "Cognitive" refers to such things as our memory, thinking, and learning. Some of the cognitive changes experienced may include these:

1. Poor concentration.
2. Becoming easily distracted.
3. Difficulty learning new information.
4. Having trouble remembering things (e.g., what someone has said earlier in the day).
5. Slowness in thought.
6. Difficulty planning.
7. Difficulty solving problems.

What is the most common change in cognitive functioning?

The most common change people notice is that they have more difficulty in remembering everyday things. This is a result of problems in short-term memory—for example, remembering the name of someone you just met or what you discussed with someone earlier in the day. Difficulties with memory may cause lowered self-confidence because people cannot remember the things that are important to the people they spend time with. Such difficulties may also cause problems at work.

Is there any way of knowing how severe the cognitive changes will be?

Generally, the more severe the injury, the more severe the cognitive difficulties that result. Research has shown that severe memory problems are more likely to occur in those who have had a posttraumatic amnesia lasting more than 7 days. However, there is a tremendous amount of individual difference. Different people are affected to a different extent by an injury of seemingly similar severity. Sometimes it is the people with mild cognitive problems who are most distressed about the change. This is particularly so if they have high expectations that can no longer be met.

How long will the cognitive changes last?

Most of the improvement in cognitive functioning occurs within 12 months of suffering a traumatic brain injury. However, some gradual improvement may continue for many years. Often, cognitive difficulties persist (e.g., memory problems, difficulty learning, or inability to concentrate). Usually, verbal skills (e.g., knowing the meaning of words, being able to correctly name objects) return to a near-normal level. Other cognitive abilities such as being able to keep concentrating on a task, or being able to remember a lot of information, are more affected by traumatic brain injury and do not recover as quickly or as completely. Like the changes in personality, changes in cognitive functioning are reported most often at around 1 year after the accident. In the early stages of recovery, they are reported more often by friends and relatives than by the traumatic brain-injured individuals themselves.

Can anything be done about these cognitive changes?

Over the years, a number of programs have been designed that attempt to improve cognitive functioning after traumatic brain injury. Typically, these programs involve the person with the traumatic brain injury practicing a number of cognitive tasks (e.g., completing puzzles or tasks on a computer). These programs do appear to help in some cases, but for many people they are not particularly successful. Sometimes these programs result in improved ability on a very specific task (e.g., remembering lists of items), but at a practical level they do not improve overall cognitive ability in everyday life. They also require a lot of time and dedication on the part of the individual and his or her friends or relatives. It may prove more useful to learn techniques to help make up for any cognitive problems. Some people can become so expert at using these techniques that their cognitive difficulties are less distressing to them. It is also important to realize that in the long term it seems to be the personality, mood, and social changes that cause the most concern.

Some Ideas for Coping with Cognitive Changes

Memory

1. Arrange set places to put easily lost objects such as keys and wallets.
2. Improve the likelihood of remembering information by learning it in as many different ways as possible (e.g., say it to yourself, write it down, and get others to remind you).
3. Repeat to yourself any important information. This helps move information into long-term memory, making recall more likely.
4. Improve memory for names and faces by pairing them with a noticeable feature about the person (e.g., Barry, bald).
5. Use daily planners or diaries.
6. Tell people you have a poor memory so they can help you.
7. Do not be overly concerned about an occasional memory lapse. We all have such lapses, and we expect others to have them too.

Learning

1. Learn in a quiet place away from distraction (e.g., TV, radio, people talking).
2. Tackle small chunks of material at a time (e.g., aim to read two pages, not a whole chapter).
3. Work for short periods of time (e.g., 10–30 minutes).
4. Get another person to demonstrate what needs to be learned, especially if it is a manual skill (e.g., how to repair a leaking tap). "Guided practice" may also improve learning. Guided practice involves a hands-on approach in which the learner attempts the task and the teacher physically guides the learner.
5. Practice the newly learned skill. There is no substitute for practice.

Neurological Changes

Neurological problems that commonly result from traumatic brain injury include difficulty with walking and balance, visual problems (usually double vision), and increased risk of epilepsy. Some people also find that they lose their sense of smell. Hearing can also be affected. Most of these changes are permanent and are a result of damage to the brain and the cranial nerves. The expert advisor in this area is your neurologist, your neurosurgeon, or your family physician. It is recommended that you consult them for further information about these changes.

SESSION 4

Social Changes

The changes in social behavior that occur after traumatic brain injury are complicated. Social behavior refers to how we get on with other people. This may be in our workplace, with friends, or at social gatherings. It also refers to the time we spend at sports or hobbies. In this session, we will look at four different areas in which social change may occur: returning to work, relationships with friends, participation in hobbies and sports, and social skills.

How many people return to work after a traumatic brain injury?

The chances of a person's returning to work depend largely on the severity of the effects of injury. Studies including very severely injured persons typically report return-to-work rates of less than 50%. Studies of moderate to severely injured individuals report return-to-work rates of between 50% and 85%. Many factors other than the severity of injury can affect whether or not a person returns to work. These factors include the employer's willingness to offer support, the availability of salary compensation, and availability of work rehabilitation services. Returning to work seems to be more difficult for those with significant cognitive problems or personality change or both.

What happens to involvement in hobbies and sports after a traumatic brain injury?

Having a traumatic brain injury can make a big difference in the number and type of leisure activities a person can engage in. Some people are advised to give up their favorite but dangerous pastimes, such as rugby, boxing, or motorcycle riding. Others find that they simply are no longer interested in engaging in hobbies or sports. A decrease in the amount of recreational activity is a very common experience following traumatic brain injury.

What causes this reduction?

It does not seem to be a result of physical problems (e.g., broken legs), but may be caused by the personality, emotional, and cognitive changes that we have talked about earlier. Changes in motivation also affect leisure activity. People with less severe injuries tend to get back to their sports and hobbies quickly, whereas those with more severe injuries are less likely to do so.

Why does it matter that sports and hobbies are dropped?

Sports and hobbies are an important part of our feeling good about life. People who take part in them are generally happier, healthier people. Sports and hobbies are good for our bodies in a physical way, and socially they give us a chance to meet people. It is very important to encourage involvement in a hobby or sport of some sort, even if it is very different from that which a person might have engaged in before his accident.

What can be done to help people get back into their sports and hobbies?

The first step is to think of a variety of activities that are enjoyable and can be done without too much hassle. Plan how to get involved in these activities (e.g., how I can learn, what I need to buy, when I can do it). Joining a club can be a good option, as it sometimes seems to be easier to get motivated in a group. Remember to avoid returning to activities with the potential of causing serious traumatic brain injury (e.g., boxing, rugby).

How do relationships with friends change after a traumatic brain injury?

A large proportion of people who have had a traumatic brain injury report that after the accident they have fewer friends and spend less time with these friends. There are also some suggestions that the quality of friendships is poorer following a traumatic brain injury.

How common is this problem?

Even for moderately injured people, problems with lack of friends are serious for approximately a third of people. This "social isolation" does tend to improve over time. However, a typical pattern is for people to lose many of their preinjury friends, but to slowly build up a new friendship network. This can be very distressing for the injured persons, their families, and their friends.

What causes the problem?

Loss of friends is not directly caused by damage to the brain, but seems to be a result of the personality changes that may occur following traumatic brain injury. The personality changes can mean that the individual acts differently in social situations, likes different things, and behaves differently with family and friends. Relationships may become less close, and in some cases most or all past friendships are lost and the person is not easily able to make new friends. This is more likely to happen if the injury is severe or the person has serious cognitive problems. Cognitive problems such as poor memory, lack of concentration, and difficulty understanding social situations make it more difficult to relate to other people.

What are social skills and how do they change?

"Social skills" is a term that covers a wide range of behaviors that are important when one person is talking with another person. It includes such things as the ability to start a conversation, take turns when talking, and laugh and smile at the right times. After a traumatic brain injury, some of these skills seem to be impaired. People may, for example, talk very little and be unable to hold a conversation, or they may talk at length about things that are not interesting to the other person. They may also speak slowly and with few changes in the tone of their voice. This can make it harder to talk with the person and makes conversations less enjoyable.

How common is the problem of decreased social skills?

These difficulties are a serious problem for over half of people with a traumatic brain injury. Often, social-skills problems are not recognized by the person himself; however, friends or relatives may notice the changes. The good news about social skills is that they may improve somewhat across time and can be relearned using social-skills training.

Why are social skills important?

The lack of social skills may be one reason that people who have experienced a traumatic brain injury lose some of their friends and no longer socialize as often. If social skills do not recover, or are not relearned, the person may not be as much fun to be with and friends simply slip away.

What can be done?

Training in social skills can help. Social-skills training involves relearning skills necessary to hold a rewarding conversation. What is learned as part of social-skills training depends very much on the person concerned.

B

Profile of Functional Impairment in Communication (PFIC)

Richard J. Linscott, Robert G. Knight, and Hamish P. D. Godfrey

OBSERVER REPORT FORM

General Information

Date: ____________________ Time: ____________________

Information source: ☐ Observation ☐ Interview ☐ Video record

Observer details: Name: ________________________
Number: ________________

Subject details: Name: ________________________

Number: ________________ Group: ________________

Age: __________ Sex: ☐ Male ☐ Female

RICHARD J. LINSCOTT, ROBERT G. KNIGHT, and HAMISH P. D. GODFREY • Department of Psychology, University of Otago, Dunedin, New Zealand.

Introductory Notes and Instructions

1. The purpose of the checklist is the detection of functional impairment in communication.
2. The context of assessment of communication impairment should be a dyadic interaction. Assessment should ideally be based on multiple interactions occurring at different times, provided that the level of structure in the interactions is homogeneous.
3. The individual whose communication is being assessed is referred to as the *subject*; the individual with whom the subject communicates in the dialogue(s) is referred to as the *other.*
4. For each section, it is important to bear in mind the aspect of the dialogue(s) being coded. This aspect is outlined at the beginning of each section.
5. Some items are asterisked. This marking is for scoring purposes. Respond to all items, *including* those that are asterisked.
6. There are 85 items and 10 summary items distributed across 10 sections. Read each item carefully, making one response for each of the 95 items. Make sure responses are clear and *not* overlapping. Make any alterations obvious.
7. Rate all items using the following scale:

   N.A. = Not applicable
   0 = Not at all
   1 = Occasionally
   2 = Often
   3 = Nearly always or always

Section 1: Logical Content

Ideal: Irrespective of context, social appropriateness, relevance, or any other contextually derived factors, an utterance should be logical and understandable.

Bear in mind what is actually said—words, grammar, syntax, and semantics—disregarding inferences that can be drawn from the context of the conversation that may add additional meaning to the utterances.

Logical Content

1.01	The flow of utterances is disrupted and broken (dysfluency).	N.A.	0	1	2	3	–
1.02	Sentences are fragmented.	N.A.	0	1	2	3	–

1.03	Uses simple sentence structures.	N.A.	0	1	2	3	–
1.04	Uses meaningless words.	N.A.	0	1	2	3	–
1.05	Describes simple things with many words (circumlocutions).	N.A.	0	1	2	3	–
1.06	Says odd or bizarre things.	N.A.	0	1	2	3	–
1.07	Says sounds or words unintentionally (paraphasic utterances).	N.A.	0	1	2	3	–
1.08	Has difficulty naming objects (anomic).	N.A.	0	1	2	3	–
1.09	Uses peculiar catchphrases.	N.A.	0	1	2	3	–
1.10	Leaves out parts of sentences.	N.A.	0	1	2	3	–

General: *Overall*, and considering the relative importance of any deficits listed in the above items, how would you rate the subject's ability to use logical, understandable, and coherent language?

- ☐ Normal
- ☐ Very mildly impaired
- ☐ Mildly impaired
- ☐ Moderately impaired
- ☐ Severely impaired
- ☐ Very severely impaired

Section 2: General Participation

Ideal: Subject contributes to a dialogue in an effort to meet an (implicit or explicit) conversational goal that has some shared value.

Bearing in mind the subject's contribution as a whole, consider the subject's coordination of ideas, attempts to meet the listener's needs, and his or her general participation.

General Participation

*2.01	Ideas are well-knit and cohesively organized.	N.A.	0	1	2	3	+
2.02	Appears disinterested in the other.	N.A.	0	1	2	3	–
*2.03	Responds to social initiatives.	N.A.	0	1	2	3	+
*2.04	Asks questions.	N.A.	0	1	2	3	+
2.05	Is boring to listen to.	N.A.	0	1	2	3	–
2.06	Gives unfriendly responses to other's social initiatives.	N.A.	0	1	2	3	–
2.07	Appears unskillful.	N.A.	0	1	2	3	–
*2.08	Contributes spontaneously to conversation.	N.A.	0	1	2	3	+
*2.09	Is skilled at taking turns.	N.A.	0	1	2	3	+
*2.10	Contributes equally to the conversation.	N.A.	0	1	2	3	+
2.11	Is dominating.	N.A.	0	1	2	3	–

2.12	Is difficult to converse with.	N.A.	0	1	2	3	–

General: *Overall*, and considering the relative importance of any deficits listed in the above items, how would you rate the subject's ability to participate in social interaction in a manner that is organized and sensitive to the other's interests?

- ☐ Normal
- ☐ Very mildly impaired
- ☐ Mildly impaired
- ☐ Moderately impaired
- ☐ Severely impaired
- ☐ Very severely impaired

Section 3: Quantity

Ideal: Information provided matches listener's needs.

Bear in mind the amount of information that the subject provides and how that level of information matches (or does not match) the other's needs.

Quantity

3.01	Talks over other's head.	N.A.	0	1	2	3	–
3.02	Provides excessive detail.	N.A.	0	1	2	3	–
*3.03	Perceives other's misinterpretation of meaning.	N.A.	0	1	2	3	+
*3.04	Is responsive to requests for clarification.	N.A.	0	1	2	3	+
3.05	Provides insufficient detail.	N.A.	0	1	2	3	–
3.06	Uses jargon inappropriately.	N.A.	0	1	2	3	–
3.07	Patronizes others.	N.A.	0	1	2	3	–

General: *Overall*, and considering the relative importance of any deficits listed in the above items, how would you rate the subject's ability to provide an appropriate amount of information given the other's needs or understanding?

- ☐ Normal
- ☐ Very mildly impaired
- ☐ Mildly impaired
- ☐ Moderately impaired
- ☐ Severely impaired
- ☐ Very severely impaired

Section 4: Quality

Ideal: Subject's contributions to conversation are true to the subject's knowledge and beliefs.

Bear in mind how honest and factual the subject's contribution appears, noting that this is *not* a character rating, but a subjective evaluation of how the subject *appears* in the situation(s) being considered.

Quality

4.01	Makes up stories (confabulates).	N.A.	0	1	2	3	–
4.02	Exaggerates.	N.A.	0	1	2	3	–
*4.03	Is consistent.	N.A.	0	1	2	3	+
*4.04	Appears to be telling the truth.	N.A.	0	1	2	3	+
4.05	Boasts.	N.A.	0	1	2	3	–

General: *Overall*, and considering the relative importance of any deficits listed in the above items, how would you rate the subject's ability to contribute information in a manner that appears honest or factual?

- ☐ Normal
- ☐ Very mildly impaired
- ☐ Mildly impaired
- ☐ Moderately impaired
- ☐ Severely impaired
- ☐ Very severely impaired

Section 5: Internal Relation

Ideal: The relationship between successive ideas within a turn at speaking should be clear and cohesive in nature; ideas should be immediately relevant and related.

Bearing in mind the subject's turns at speaking in isolation from the other's turns, consider the structuring and the relatedness of the ideas the subject presents.

Internal Relation

5.01	Overuses elaboration.	N.A.	0	1	2	3	–
*5.02	There is good continuity between ideas.	N.A.	0	1	2	3	+
5.03	Overemphasizes unimportant ideas.	N.A.	0	1	2	3	–
5.04	Repeats information.	N.A.	0	1	2	3	–
5.05	Deemphasizes central ideas.	N.A.	0	1	2	3	–
5.06	Ideas appear jumbled or poorly coordinated.	N.A.	0	1	2	3	–
*5.07	Elaborates spontaneously.	N.A.	0	1	2	3	+
5.08	Ideas are illogically connected (thought-disordered).	N.A.	0	1	2	3	–

General: *Overall*, and considering the relative importance of any deficits listed in the above items, how would you rate the subject's ability to contribute ideas in an organized and related manner?

- ☐ Normal
- ☐ Very mildly impaired
- ☐ Mildly impaired
- ☐ Moderately impaired
- ☐ Severely impaired
- ☐ Very severely impaired

Section 6: External Relation

Ideal: There is a good relation between the ideas presented in a turn at speaking and the ideas presented by the other's immediately preceding turn.

Bear in mind the relation and relevance between the subject's turns and the other's turns. [Note that items related to questions assume that questions were asked (see item 2.04). If they were not, mark as not applicable.]

External Relation

*6.01	Gives responses to listener (e.g., "... right ... yeah ... mmm, is that so? ... aha ...").	N.A.	0	1	2	3	+
6.02	Mimics other's utterances (echolalia).	N.A.	0	1	2	3	–
*6.03	Gives appropriate types of listener responses.	N.A.	0	1	2	3	+
6.04	Asks inappropriate questions.	N.A.	0	1	2	3	–
*6.05	Uses questions well.	N.A.	0	1	2	3	+
*6.06	Integrates own ideas with other's ideas.	N.A.	0	1	2	3	+

General: *Overall*, and considering the relative importance of any deficits listed in the above items, how would you rate the subject's ability to relate his or her own comments to the other's preceding contributions?

- ☐ Normal
- ☐ Very mildly impaired
- ☐ Mildly impaired
- ☐ Moderately impaired
- ☐ Severely impaired
- ☐ Very severely impaired

Section 7: Clarity of Expression

Ideal: Ideas are presented clearly.

Bear in mind the conciseness with which ideas are presented, disregarding dysfluency or articulation problems that the subject might exhibit.

Clarity of Expression

7.01	Is ambiguous or vague.	N.A.	0	1	2	3	–
*7.02	Uses lucid, clear, or succinct expression.	N.A.	0	1	2	3	+
7.03	Is obscure.	N.A.	0	1	2	3	–

General: *Overall*, and considering the relative importance of any deficits listed in the above items, how would you rate the subject's ability to express ideas clearly and concisely?	☐ Normal ☐ Very mildly impaired ☐ Mildly impaired ☐ Moderately impaired ☐ Severely impaired ☐ Very severely impaired

Section 8: Social Style

Ideal: Contributions to a conversation should be appropriate given the context and background of the conversation and the subject's relationship with the other.

Bear in mind the context of the conversation and how the subject's style matches the context, irrespective of the topic of the conversation.

Social Style

8.01	Is overpolite or overcourteous.	N.A.	0	1	2	3	–
8.02	Gives excessive attention.	N.A.	0	1	2	3	–
8.03	Is overly respectful or flattering toward the other.	N.A.	0	1	2	3	–
8.04	Is too informal.	N.A.	0	1	2	3	–
8.05	Dominates control over conversational direction.	N.A.	0	1	2	3	–
8.06	Is overly formal or ceremonious.	N.A.	0	1	2	3	–
*8.07	Helps direct the conversation.	N.A.	0	1	2	3	+
8.08	Is impolite or discourteous.	N.A.	0	1	2	3	–
8.09	Gives inappropriate types of attention.	N.A.	0	1	2	3	–
8.10	Pays insufficient attention.	N.A.	0	1	2	3	–
8.11	Shows disrespect or irreverence toward the other.	N.A.	0	1	2	3	–

General: *Overall*, and considering the relative importance of any deficits listed in the above items, how would you rate the subject's ability to use an appropriate social style?	☐ Normal ☐ Very mildly impaired ☐ Mildly impaired ☐ Moderately impaired ☐ Severely impaired ☐ Very severely impaired

Section 9: Subject Matter

Ideal: The topic content should be appropriate given the moral, cultural, and social background and values of the context and the other.

Bear in mind what the subject has actually said, and the appropriateness of what was said, especially in terms of offensiveness or deviance, given the social and cultural context.

Subject Matter

9.01	Is overly intimate.	N.A.	0	1	2	3	–
9.02	Inappropriate (sexual, religious, political) content.	N.A.	0	1	2	3	–
9.03	Talks about self too much (egocentric).	N.A.	0	1	2	3	–
9.04	Uses profanity or obscenity.	N.A.	0	1	2	3	–
9.05	Is abusive or insulting to self or other.	N.A.	0	1	2	3	–

General: *Overall*, and considering the relative importance of any deficits listed in the above items, how would you rate the subject's ability to adhere to socially, culturally, or morally appropriate subject matter in conversations?

- ☐ Normal
- ☐ Very mildly impaired
- ☐ Mildly impaired
- ☐ Moderately impaired
- ☐ Severely impaired
- ☐ Very severely impaired

Section 10: Aesthetics

Ideal: A certain level of quantitative and qualitative aesthetic variation is used to add meaning, emphasis, or variety to the contribution made by the participants.

Bear in mind the subject's interaction as a whole; when the method of observation precludes ascertainment of the particular behavior, rate as not applicable.

Aesthetics

10.01	Has a long response latency.	N.A.	0	1	2	3	–
10.02	Voice is too loud.	N.A.	0	1	2	3	–
10.03	Speaks too rapidly.	N.A.	0	1	2	3	–
10.04	Speaks in monotone voice.	N.A.	0	1	2	3	–
10.05	Is restless and fidgety.	N.A.	0	1	2	3	–
10.06	Interrupts.	N.A.	0	1	2	3	–
10.07	Performs inappropriate grooming behaviors during conversation.	N.A.	0	1	2	3	–
10.08	Uses humor inappropriately.	N.A.	0	1	2	3	–
10.09	Speaks too slowly.	N.A.	0	1	2	3	–
*10.10	Uses affective expression appropriately.	N.A.	0	1	2	3	+

10.11	Voice is pitched excessively high or low.	N.A.	0	1	2	3	–
10.12	Scratches self.	N.A.	0	1	2	3	–
10.13	Speaks too softly.	N.A.	0	1	2	3	–
10.14	Speech contains long or many pauses.	N.A.	0	1	2	3	–
*10.15	Articulates words clearly.	N.A.	0	1	2	3	+
10.16	Uses unusual or excessive gesturing.	N.A.	0	1	2	3	–
10.17	Uses wordplay inappropriately.	N.A.	0	1	2	3	–
*10.18	Uses normal phoneme stress.	N.A.	0	1	2	3	+

General: *Overall*, and considering the relative importance of any deficits listed in the above items, how would you rate the subject's ability to color his or her contribution to social interaction with aesthetic features?

- ☐ Normal
- ☐ Very mildly impaired
- ☐ Mildly impaired
- ☐ Moderately impaired
- ☐ Severely impaired
- ☐ Very severely impaired

C

Summary of Intervention Strategies

COGNITIVE IMPAIRMENT

Memory impairment

(a) Use of external compensatory aids
(b) Use of internal compensatory techniques
(c) Social-skills training

Poor concentration

(a) Alternating tasks with high and low cognitive demands
(b) Restricting the number of tasks carried out simultaneously

Difficulty learning new information

(a) Teaching learning strategies
(b) Guided practice

Impaired problem-solving and decision-making ability

(a) Problem-solving training
(b) Prioritization skills

Planning disorders

(a) Self-instructional training
(b) Use of checklists

EMOTIONAL ADJUSTMENT

Anxiety

(a) Relaxation training
(b) Activity scheduling
(c) Graduated exposure
(d) Cognitive strategies
(e) Risk minimization

Depression

(a) Cognitive strategies
(b) Behavioral strategies
(c) Preventative strategies

Grief

(a) Reenactment and expression of feelings
(b) Graduated exposure

Negative self-concept

(a) "New you" concept
(b) Improving self-appraisal

Irritability

(a) Avoiding trigger situations
(b) Environmental modification
(c) Teaching coping responses
(d) Family education

Catastrophic reactions

(a) Education
(b) Crisis intervention
(c) Liaison with family members and health professionals

Lack of awareness

(a) Education
(b) Hierarchical questioning
(c) Feedback
(d) Planned "self-discovery"

SOCIAL COMPETENCY

Impaired interpersonal skills

(a) Interpersonal-skills training

Low rates of social interaction

(a) Education
(b) Goal setting
(c) Cognitive strategies

Low rates of participation in leisure pursuits

(a) Education
(b) Problem solving
(c) Goal setting

Vocational adjustment

(a) Vocational assessment
(b) Prevocational training
(c) Vocational placement

BEHAVIORAL FUNCTIONING

Behavioral excesses
- (a) Education
- (b) Antecedent control techniques
- (c) Contingency management
- (d) Cognitive strategies

Addictive behaviors
- (a) Education
- (b) Review of negative consequences
- (c) Avoidance of trigger situations
- (d) Prescheduled alternate activities
- (e) Social support
- (f) Contingency management
- (g) Relapse prevention

Behavioral deficits
- (a) Self-instructional training
- (b) Goal setting
- (c) Contingency management

FAMILY ADAPTATION

Lack of knowledge
- (a) Education program

Strained family relationships
- (a) Support
- (b) Expression of feelings
- (c) Scheduled pleasant activities
- (d) Communication-skills training
- (e) Problem-solving training
- (f) Cognitive strategies

Demands on caregiver
- (a) Accessing community resources
- (b) Crisis intervention services
- (c) Support
- (d) Case monitoring
- (e) Providing emotional support
- (f) Respite care
- (g) Attendant care
- (h) Teaching behavior management skills
- (i) Support groups

D

Case-by-Case Matching

Demographic and Injury Variables[a]

Group	Name	Age	Marital status	Education (years)	LOH (days)	PTA (days)	GCS	N. Int.?
E	Susan	28	Married	12	11	NA	NA	Yes
C	Matthew	43	Married	10	16	9	9	Yes
E	Richard	20	Single	12	70	31	6	No
C	Daniel	21	Married	11	66	31	5	No
E	Brian	17	Single	12	8	5	13	No
C	Mary	18	Single	11	2	7	7	No
E	Graham	31	Single	11	18	10	NA	No
C	Paul	33	Single	11	25	10	12	Yes
E	Keith	26	Single	11	29	14	10	No
C	Mark	17	Single	11	25	14	11	No
E	Grant	27	Married	12	17	10	12	No
C	John	19	Single	14	14	7	13	No
E	Hamish	34	Married	12	5	2	14	No
C	Joshua	20	Married	12	3	3	13	No
E	Joseph	17	Single	12	36	23	6	No
C	David	23	Single	11	56	10	8	No
E	Aaron	19	Single	11	52	28	6	No
C	Adam	23	Single	16	51	14	9	No
E	Patrick	36	Single	10	16	18	9	No
C	Michael	36	Single	10	23	14	6	No
E	Peter	28	Single	14	35	28	11	No
C	Andrew	16	Single	11	84	32	6	Yes
E	Derek	29	Single	11	56	30	4	Yes
C	Margaret	20	Single	10	82	NA	7	No
E	Simon	37	Married	11	31	6	13	No
C	Peter	28	Single	15	54	10	13	No

(Continued)

Group	Name	Age	Marital status	Education (years)	LOH (days)	PTA (days)	GCS	N. Int.?
E	Annette	17	Single	10	10	4	9	No
C	Thomas	26	Single	11	9	NA	13	No

[a]Group: E = experimental, C = control; LOH = length of hospitalization; PTA = length of posttraumatic amnesia; GCS = Glasgow Coma Scale score on admission; N. Int.? = neurosurgical intervention required?; NA = data not available.

Cognitive Variables[a]

Group	Name	NART	RAVLT	RPM	MH	COWAT	PASAT	MMS
E	Susan	98	70	100	85	49	25	26
C	Matthew	92	67	111	81	43	28	29
E	Richard	114	25	102	95	18	9	28
C	Daniel	106	53	96	91	40	24	29
E	Brian	102	64	108	98	33	27	28
C	Mary	111	81	118	102	42	48	30
E	Graham	104	53	125	90	48	54	30
C	Paul	120	59	130	110	59	56	29
E	Keith	103	53	98	85	35	48	30
C	Mark	92	44	97	85	26	25	28
E	Grant	112	36	101	96	45	37	28
C	John	110	83	115	101	41	50	30
E	Hamish	113	68	125	99	48	46	30
C	Joshua	112	36	101	96	45	37	28
E	Joseph	101	47	110	89	15	24	29
C	David	88	50	102	77	27	NA	27
E	Aaron	93	70	93	91	31	16	28
C	Adam	111	76	118	92	43	55	29
E	Patrick	97	42	104	91	43	28	28
C	Michael	97	57	101	93	34	11	24
E	Peter	119	66	104	102	54	33	30
C	Andrew	86	48	75	88	28	0	24
E	Derek	100	55	96	96	29	22	26
C	Margaret	89	21	66	76	10	18	23
E	Simon	104	60	110	93	38	34	29
C	Peter	121	59	108	91	50	54	30
E	Annette	89	60	94	89	19	33	26
C	Thomas	NA	NA	NA	NA	NA	NA	NA

[a]Group: E = experimental, C = control; NART = National Adult Reading Test; RAVLT = Rey Auditory Verbal Learning Test; RPM = Ravens Standard Progressive Matrices; MH = Mill Hill Vocabulary Scale; COWAT = Controlled Oral Word Association Test; PASAT = Paced Auditory Serial-Addition Task; MMS = Mini Mental State exam; NA = data not available.

E

Head Injury Behavior Scale

Patient Version: To be completed by the head injury sufferer.

INSTRUCTIONS: Below is a list of problem behaviors that you may be experiencing. Please indicate whether each of the behaviors listed is a problem *for you* by circling Yes or No as appropriate. For each problem behavior circled Yes, please indicate how much distress the behavior causes you by circling a number on the scale (1–4). Remember, we are asking you to report about your own behavior, *not* the behavior of others. Use the following rating scale:

Head Injury Behavior Rating Scale

1. The behavior is a problem for me but causes me *no* distress.
2. The behavior is a problem for me and causes me *mild* distress.
3. The behavior is a problem for me and causes me *moderate* distress.
4. The behavior is a problem for me and causes me *severe* distress.

Behavior	Is the behavior a *problem*?		How much *distress* does the problem cause?			
1. Anger; difficulty controlling temper.	Yes	No	1	2	3	4
2. Impatient; upset when needs not easily met.	Yes	No	1	2	3	4
3. Frequent complaining.	Yes	No	1	2	3	4
4. Aggression; violent behavior.	Yes	No	1	2	3	4
5. Impulsivity; do things without thinking.	Yes	No	1	2	3	4
6. Argumentative; often dispute topics.	Yes	No	1	2	3	4

7. Lack control over behavior; behavior is inappropriate for social situations.	Yes	No	1	2	3	4
8. Overly dependent; rely on others unnecessarily; do not do things for myself.	Yes	No	1	2	3	4
9. Poor decision making; do not think of consequences.	Yes	No	1	2	3	4
10. Childish; at times behavior is immature.	Yes	No	1	2	3	4
11. Poor insight; refuse to admit difficulties.	Yes	No	1	2	3	4
12. Difficulty in becoming interested in things.	Yes	No	1	2	3	4
13. Lack of initiative; do not think for myself.	Yes	No	1	2	3	4
14. Irritable; snappy; grumpy.	Yes	No	1	2	3	4
15. Sudden/rapid mood change.	Yes	No	1	2	3	4
16. Anxious; tense; uptight.	Yes	No	1	2	3	4
17. Depressed; low mood.	Yes	No	1	2	3	4
18. Irresponsible; can't always be trusted.	Yes	No	1	2	3	4
19. Overly sensitive; easily upset.	Yes	No	1	2	3	4
20. Lack motivation; lack of interest in doing things.	Yes	No	1	2	3	4

Relative/Friend Version: To be completed by a relative or friend of the sufferer.

INSTRUCTIONS: Below is a list of problem behaviors the sufferer may be experiencing. Please indicate whether each of the behaviors listed is a problem for the sufferer by circling Yes or No as appropriate. For each problem behavior circled Yes, please indicate how much distress the behavior causes *you* by circling a number on the scale (1–4). Remember, we are asking you to report about the sufferer's behavior. Use the following scale:

Head Injury Behavior Rating Scale

1. The behavior is a problem for sufferer but causes me *no* distress.
2. The behavior is a problem for sufferer and causes me *mild* distress.
3. The behavior is a problem for sufferer and causes me *moderate* distress.
4. The behavior is a problem for sufferer and causes me *severe* distress.

Behavior	Is the behavior a *problem*?		How much *distress* does the problem cause?			
1. Anger; difficulty controlling temper.	Yes	No	1	2	3	4
2. Impatient; upset when needs not easily met.	Yes	No	1	2	3	4
3. Frequent complaining.	Yes	No	1	2	3	4
4. Aggression; violent behavior.	Yes	No	1	2	3	4
5. Impulsivity; does things without thinking.	Yes	No	1	2	3	4
6. Argumentative; often disputes topics.	Yes	No	1	2	3	4
7. Lacks control over behavior; behavior is inappropriate for social situations.	Yes	No	1	2	3	4
8. Overly dependent; relies on others unnecessarily; does not do things for him/herself.	Yes	No	1	2	3	4
9. Poor decision making; does not think of consequences.	Yes	No	1	2	3	4
10. Childish; at times behavior is immature.	Yes	No	1	2	3	4
11. Poor insight; refuses to admit difficulties.	Yes	No	1	2	3	4
12. Difficulty in becoming interested in things.	Yes	No	1	2	3	4
13. Lack of initiative; does not think for him/herself.	Yes	No	1	2	3	4
14. Irritable; snappy; grumpy.	Yes	No	1	2	3	4
15. Sudden/rapid mood change.	Yes	No	1	2	3	4
16. Anxious; tense; uptight.	Yes	No	1	2	3	4
17. Depressed; low mood.	Yes	No	1	2	3	4
18. Irresponsible; can't always be trusted.	Yes	No	1	2	3	4
19. Overly sensitive; easily upset.	Yes	No	1	2	3	4
20. Lacks motivation; lack of interest in doing things.	Yes	No	1	2	3	4

F

Results of the Consumer Satisfaction Questionnaire

	Not at all		Moderately so			Very much so	
Scale:	1	2	3	4	5	6	7

Question	Respondents	Mean	SD
To what extent was the advice given by the psychologist helpful?	Patients	6.3	1.3
	Relatives	6.5	0.8
To what extent has receiving the service helped your adjustment to head injury?	Patients	5.8	1.5
	Relatives	—	—
To what extent do you think that being in the service has improved [patient's] adjustment to head injury?	Patients	—	—
	Relatives	6.6	0.7
To what extent do you think that being in the service helped you deal better with [patient's] head injury?	Patients	—	—
	Relatives	6.6	0.6
To what extent was meeting in your home preferable to hospital appointments?	Patients	6.5	1.0
	Relatives	6.9	0.3
To what extent was it helpful to have ongoing contact with the psychologist throughout the 18 months?	Patients	6.5	0.8
	Relatives	6.7	0.6
Were you happy with the number of visits you received?	Patients	5.9	1.2
	Relatives	6.4	1.3
To what extent did you feel that your situation was understood by the psychologist?	Patients	6.4	1.0
	Relatives	6.3	1.1
To what extent did you receive adequate emotional support and reassurance?	Patients	5.4	1.3
	Relatives	5.9	1.1
To what extent do you think that you received adequate education about head injury and its consequences?	Patients	6.1	1.0
	Relatives	6.3	0.9
To what extent was the educational material easy to follow?	Patients	5.2	1.3
	Relatives	5.9	1.7
To what extent was having someone discussing the education with you helpful?	Patients	6.4	0.9
	Relatives	6.4	1.6
To what extent do you think that the education you received improved the way you dealt with head injury?	Patients	5.2	1.6
	Relatives	5.6	1.1

G

Case Management Assessment Areas

Social Contact

How many times has the TBI individual gone out to a social event in the past two weeks?
How many visitors has the TBI individual received in the past two weeks?
How frequently has the TBI individual participated in leisure activities?
Is the TBI individual displaying interpersonal-skills deficits?
What are the factors that interfere with the TBI individual's participation in social activity?
Is the TBI individual attempting to pursue social activities that are now unsafe because of the risk of reinjury?
Are goals for social activity being met?
Has the TBI individual experienced conflict in any close relationships, particularly with partner or parents?
What, if anything, has the TBI individual done to increase the partner's satisfaction with their relationship?
Are there any difficulties in the TBI individual's sexual relationship?
Is the TBI individual able to communicate adequately with family and friends?

Work Performance

How many hours has the TBI individual worked in the past two weeks?
What is the exact nature of the task he or she is undertaking?
Is the TBI individual attending work punctually, and on a regular basis?
Is the TBI individual satisfied with the work placement? If not, why not?
How long can the TBI individual work before becoming fatigued?
Is the TBI individual able to socialize with workmates at tea breaks and lunchtimes?

What are the TBI individual's expectations regarding his or her work performance?
Have arrangements been made to teach the TBI individual new skills relevant to his or her job?
Is the TBI individual receiving feedback from an employer or supervisor with respect to his or her work performance?
Is the TBI individual able to complete the task that has been assigned?
Are there any alterations to the work environment that need to be made?
What compensatory strategies is the TBI individual utilizing within the work environment?
What is the TBI individual's appraisal of his or her own work performance?

Cognitive Functioning

How long can the TBI individual attend to a complex task as compared with a simple task?
What factors cause the TBI individual's attention to decrease?
Is the TBI individual displaying signs of memory impairment?
Is neuropsychological testing required?
Are compensatory strategies being employed? If not, why not?
Has the TBI individual had to learn new information in the past two weeks?
If so, was he or she able to learn the information?
What decisions has the TBI individual made in the past two weeks? Review these decisions with the TBI individual.
Utilize the problem-solving format to address with the TBI individual any problems that may have arisen.

Mood Disturbance

Is the TBI individual demonstrating signs of depression?
How frequent and intense are depressive episodes?
Has there been suicidal ideation or a suicide attempt?
Have there been changes in the TBI individual's eating and sleeping patterns?
Does the TBI individual report ruminating on what life was like before the accident?
Is the TBI individual meeting his or her performance expectations?
What is the TBI individual's level of motivation?
Are there any signs of anxiety?
Is the TBI individual avoiding certain situations or events?
Is the TBI individual expressing anger, guilt, or grief about the accident?
Does the TBI individual possess an adequate self-concept?
Is the TBI individual aware of his or her deficits?

How often is the TBI individual receiving feedback on the strengths and weaknesses in his or her performance?
Have any catastrophic reactions occurred? If so, how were they handled?
Are there family members or friends that the TBI individual can discuss his or her feelings with?

Behavioral Functioning

What behavioral excesses are demonstrated by the TBI individual?
What behavioral deficits are demonstrated by the TBI individual?
Does the TBI individual possess the skills that are necessary to have his or her needs met in an appropriate manner?
Does the TBI individual demonstrate adequate daily living skills?
Is the TBI individual able to initiate and complete tasks?
Is the TBI individual aware of the "trigger" situations that precipitate aggressive behavior?
How much alcohol and drugs is the TBI individual consuming?
Are there any aspects of the TBI individual's behavior that may result in physical harm to himself or herself or to others?
Does the family have access to an alternative living arrangement for the TBI individual should his or her behavior become unmanageable?
What areas of adjustment is the TBI individual's behavior interfering with?
How are friends, family, and workmates responding to the TBI individual's behavior?

Family Coping

Do family members have support from friends and family?
Are the family having breaks away from the TBI individual?
Have the family reduced their own level of social contact in order to care for the TBI individual?
Are family members displaying signs of depression or anxiety?
Have the family received all the community services they are entitled to?
Do the family have any questions about the TBI individual's progress or about TBI in general?
Are the TBI individual's children displaying any signs of distress?
Does the family have sufficient resources to assist the TBI individual's rehabilitation?
Are the family presenting any barriers to the TBI individual's rehabilitation? If so, why?
What is the partner's long-term commitment to the relationship?

Do the family perceive that they, and the TBI individual, are receiving good service from health professionals?

Are the family aware of the impairments displayed by the TBI individual?

Do the family have realistic expectations about the TBI individual's abilities and prognosis?

References

Adamovich, B. B., Henderson, J. A., & Auerbach, S. (1985). *Cognitive rehabilitation of closed head injury patients: A dynamic approach.* San Diego, CA: College Hill Press.

Alderman, N. (1991). The treatment of avoidance behavior following severe brain injury by satiation through negative practice. *Brain Injury, 5,* 77–86.

Allen, C. C., & Ruff, R. M. (1990). Self-rating versus neuropsychological performance of moderate versus severe head injured patients. *Brain Injury, 4,* 7–17.

Anderson, J., & Parente, F. (1985). Training family members to work with the head injured patient. *Cognitive Rehabilitation,* July–August, 12–15.

Askensay, J. J., & Rahmani, L. (1988). Neuropsychosocial rehabilitation of head injury. *American Journal of Physical Medicine, 66,* 315–327.

Baddeley, A., Meade, T., & Newcombe, F. (1980). Design problems in research on rehabilitation after brain damage. *International Rehabilitation Medicine, 2,* 138–142.

Bandura, A. (1977). Self-efficacy: Toward a unifying theory of behavioral change. *Psychological Review, 84,* 191–215.

Barry, P., & Riley, J. M. (1987). Adult norms for the Kaufman Hand Movements Test and a single subject design for acute brain injury rehabilitation. *Journal of Clinical and Experimental Neuropsychology, 9,* 449–455.

Beck, A. T., & Emery, G. (1985). *Anxiety disorders and phobias: A cognitive perspective.* New York: Basic Books.

Becker, B. (1975). Intellectual changes after closed head injury. *Journal of Clinical Psychology, 31,* 307–309.

Benedict, R. H. (1989). The effectiveness of cognitive remediation strategies for victims of traumatic head injury: A review of the literature. *Clinical Psychology Review, 9,* 605–626.

Benton, A. L., & Hamsher, K. (Eds.) (1978). *The multilingual-aphasia examination.* Iowa City: University of Iowa.

Ben-Yishay, Y., & Lakin, P. (1989). Structured group treatment for brain injury survivors. In D. Ellis & A. L. Christensen (Eds.), *Neuropsychological treatment after brain injury* (pp. 271–296). Boston: Kluver Academic Publishers.

Ben-Yishay, Y., Piasetsky, E. B., & Rattok, J. (1987a). A systematic method for ameliorating disorders in basic attention. In M. J. Meier, A. L. Benton, & L. Diller (Eds.), *Neuropsychological rehabilitation* (pp. 165–182). New York: Churchill Livingstone.

Ben-Yishay, Y., Rattok, J., Lakin, P., Piasetsky, E. B., Ross, B., Silver, S., Zide, E., & Ezrachi, O. (1985). Neuropsychic rehabilitation: Quest for a holistic approach. *Seminars in Neurology, 5,* 252–259.

Ben-Yishay, Y., Silver, S. M., Piasetsky, E., & Rattok, J. (1987b). Relationship between employability and vocational outcome after intensive holistic cognitive rehabilitation. *Journal of Head Trauma Rehabilitation, 2*, 35–48.

Berrol, S. (1990). Issues in cognitive rehabilitation. *Archives of Neurology, 47*, 219–222.

Bishara, S. N., Partridge, F. M., Godfrey, H. P. D., & Knight, R. G. (1992). Post-traumatic amnesia and Glasgow Coma Scale related to outcome in survivors in a consecutive series of patients with severe closed head injury. *Brain Injury, 6*, 373–380.

Blackerby, W. F. (1990). A treatment model for sexuality disturbance following brain injury. *Journal of Head Trauma Rehabilitation, 5*, 73–82.

Boake, C., Freeland, J., Reinghalz, G., Nance, M., & Edwards, K. (1987). Awareness of memory loss after severe head injury (abstract). *Journal of Clinical and Experimental Neuropsychology, 9*, 53.

Bowers, T. G., & Clum, G. A. (1988). Relative contribution of specific and nonspecific treatment effects: Meta-analysis of placebo controlled behavior therapy research. *Psychological Bulletin, 103*, 315–323.

Brasted, W. S., & Callahan, E. J. (1984). Review article: A behavioral analysis of the grief process. *Behavior Therapy, 15*, 529–543.

Braun, C. M., Baribeau, J. M., & Ethier, M. (1988). A prospective investigation comparing patients' and relatives' symptom reports before and after a rehabilitation program for severe closed head injury. *Journal of Neurologic Rehabilitation, 2*, 109–115.

Braunling-McMorrow, D., Lloyd, K., & Fralish, K. (1986). Teaching social skills to head injured adults. *Journal of Rehabilitation, January–March*, 39–44.

Broadbent, D. E. (1958). *Decision and stress*. London: Academic Press.

Brooke, M. M., Barbour, P. G., Cording, L. G., Tolan, C., Bhoomkar, A., McCall, G. W., Lyons, C., Hudson, J., & Johnson, S. J. (1989). Nutritional status during rehabilitation after head injury. *Journal of Neurologic Rehabilitation, 3*, 27–33.

Brooks, D. N. (Ed.) (1984). *Closed head injury: Psychological, social, and family consequences*. Oxford: Oxford University Press.

Brooks, D. N. (1988). Behavioral abnormalities in head injured patients. *Scandinavian Journal of Rehabilitation Medicine, Suppl. 17*, 41–46.

Brooks, D. N. (1991). The head injured family. *Journal of Clinical and Experimental Neuropsychology, 13*, 155–188.

Brooks, D. N., & Aughton, M. E. (1979). Cognitive recovery during the first year after severe blunt head injury. *International Rehabilitation Medicine, 1*, 166–172.

Brooks, N., Campsie, L., Symington, C., Beattie, A., & McKinlay, W. (1986). The five year outcome of severe blunt head injury: A relative's view. *Journal of Neurology, Neurosurgery and Psychiatry, 49*, 764–770.

Brooks, N., Campsie, L., Symington, C., Beattie, A., & McKinlay, W. (1987a). The effects of severe head injury on patients and relatives within seven years of injury. *Journal of Head Trauma Rehabilitation, 2*, 1–13.

Brooks, N., & McKinlay, W. (1983). Personality and behavioral change after severe blunt head injury, a relative's view. *Journal of Neurology, Neurosurgery and Psychiatry, 46*, 336–344.

Brooks, N., McKinlay, W., Symington, C., Beattie, A., & Campsie, L. (1987b). Return to work within the first seven years of severe head injury. *Brain Injury, 1*, 5–19.

Brotherton, F. A., Thomas, L. L., Wisotzek, I. E., & Milan, M. A. (1988). Social skills training in the rehabilitation of patients with traumatic closed head injury. *Archives of Physical Medicine and Rehabilitation, 69*, 827–832.

Burke, W. H., & Lewis, F. D. (1986). Management of maladaptive social behavior of a brain injured adult. *International Journal of Rehabilitation Research, 9*, 335–342.

Burke, W. H., & Wesolowski, M. D. (1988). Applied behavior analysis in head injury rehabilitation. *Rehabilitation Nursing, 13*, 186–188.

Burke, W. H., Wesolowski, M. D., & Guth, M. L. (1988a). Comprehensive head injury rehabilitation: An outcome evaluation. *Brain Injury, 2*, 313–322.
Burke, W. H., Wesolowski, M. D., & Lane, I. (1988b). A positive approach to the treatment of aggressive brain injured clients. *International Journal of Rehabilitation Research, 11*, 235–241.
Burke, W. H., Zencius, A. H., Wesolowski, M. D., & Doubleday, F. (1991). Improving executive function disorders in brain injured clients. *Brain Injury, 5*, 241–252.
Butler, G. (1989). Phobic disorders. In K. Hawton, P. M. Salkovskis, J. Kirk, & D. M. Clark (Eds.), *Cognitive behavior therapy for psychiatric problems: A practical guide* (pp. 97–128). Oxford: Oxford University Press.
Campbell, D. T., & Stanley, J. C. (1966). *Experimental and quasi-experimental designs for research.* Boston: Houghton Mifflin.
Cancelliere, A. E., Moncada, C., & Reid, D. T. (1991). Memory retraining to support educational reintegration. *Archives of Physical and Medical Rehabilitation, 72*, 148–151.
Cantini, E., Gluck, M., & McLean, A. (1992). Psychotropic-absent behavioral improvement following severe traumatic brain injury. *Brain Injury, 6*, 193–197.
Christensen, A. L., Pinner, E. M., Moller Pedersen, P., Teasdale, T. W., & Trexler, L. E. (1992). Psychosocial outcome following individualized neuropsychological rehabilitation of brain damage. *Acta Neurologica Scandinavica, 85*, 32–38.
Cicerone, K. D. (1989). Psychotherapeutic interventions with traumatically brain-injured patients. *Rehabilitation Psychology, 34*, 105–114 (cf. Rosenthal, 1989).
Cicerone, K. D., & Wood, J. C. (1987). Planning disorder after closed head injury: A case study. *Archives of Physical and Medical Rehabilitation, 68*, 111–115.
Cole, J. R., Cope, N., & Cervelli, L. (1985). Rehabilitation of the severely brain-injured patient: A community-based, low cost model program. *Archives of Physical and Medical Rehabilitation, 66*, 38–40.
Cope, D. N. (1985). Traumatic closed head injury: Status of rehabilitation treatment. *Seminars in Neurology, 5*(3), 212–219.
Cope, D. N. (1987). Psychopharmacologic considerations in the treatment of traumatic brain injury. *Journal of Head Injury Rehabilitation, 2*, 1–5.
Cope, D. N., Cole, J. R., Hall, K. M., & Barkan, H. (1991a). Brain injury: Analysis of outcome in a post acute rehabilitation system. Part 1. General analysis. *Brain Injury, 5*, 111–125.
Cope, D. N., Cole, J. R., Hall, K. M., & Barkan, H. (1991b). Brain injury: Analysis of outcome in a post acute rehabilitation system. Part 2. Subanalyses. *Brain Injury, 5*, 127–139.
Cope, D. N., & Hall, K. (1982). Head injury rehabilitation: Benefit of early intervention. *Archives of Physical and Medical Rehabilitation, 63*, 433–437.
Craine, J. F. (1982). The retraining of frontal lobe dysfunction. In L. Trexler (Ed.), *Cognitive rehabilitation: Conceptualization and intervention* (pp. 229–263). New York: Plenum Press.
Cripe, L. I. (1989). Neuropsychological and psychosocial assessment of the brain injured person: Clinical concepts and guidelines. *Rehabilitation Psychology, 34*, 91–100.
Crosson, B., Novack, T. A., Trenerry, M. R., & Craig, P. L. (1988). California Verbal Learning Test (CVLT) performance in severely head-injured and neurologically normal adult males. *Journal of Clinical and Experimental Neuropsychology, 10*, 754–768.
Crowe, S. F. (1992). Dissociation of two frontal lobe syndromes by a test of verbal fluency. *Journal of Clinical and Experimental Neuropsychology, 14*, 327–339.
Deacon, D., & Campbell, K. B. (1991). Decision-making following closed head injury: Can response speed be retrained? *Journal of Clinical and Experimental Neuropsychology, 13*, 639–651.
Deaton, A. V. (1986). Denial in the aftermath of traumatic head injury: Its manifestations, measurement and treatment. *Rehabilitation Psychology, 31*, 231–240.
DeBoskey, D. S., & Morin, K. (1985). *A "how to handle" manual for families of the brain injured.* Tampa: Tampa General Rehabilitation Center.

DeFazio, A., Kelly, M. P., & Flynn, J. P. (1989). The head injured outpatient: Presentations and rehabilitation. *Maryland Medical Journal, 38*, 1035–1041.

DePoy, E. (1987). Community based occupational therapy with a head injured adult. *American Journal of Occupational Therapy, 41*, 461–464.

Diller, L. (1989). Response to "Cognitive remediation following traumatic brain injury." *Rehabilitation Psychology, 34*, 130–133 (cf. Kreutzer et al., 1989).

Dinan, T. G., & Mobayed, M. (1992). Treatment resistance of depression after head injury: A preliminary study of amitriptyline response. *Acta Psychiatrica Scandinavica, 85*, 292–294.

Durgin, C. J. (1989). Techniques for families to increase their involvement in the rehabilitation process. *Cognitive Rehabilitation, May–June*, 22–25.

Dye, O. A., Saxon, S. A., & Milby, J. B. (1981). Long term neuropsychological deficits after traumatic head injury with comatosis. *Journal of Clinical Psychology, 37*, 472–477.

D'Zurilla, T. J., & Goldfried, M. R. (1971). Problem solving and behavior modification. *Journal of Abnormal Psychology, 78*, 107–126.

Eames, P. (1992). Long term head injury problems. *Current Opinion in Neurology and Neurosurgery, 5*, 11–15.

Eames, P., & Wood, R. (1984). Rehabilitation after head injury: A special unit approach to behavior disorders. *International Rehabilitation Medicine, 7*, 130–133.

Eames, P., & Wood, R. (1985). Rehabilitation after severe brain injury: A follow-up study of a behavior modification approach. *Journal of Neurology, Neurosurgery and Psychiatry, 48*, 613–619.

Editorial (1990). Head trauma victims in the UK: Undeservedly underserved. *Lancet, 335*, 886–887.

Eisner, J., & Kreutzer, J. E. (1989). A family information system for education following traumatic brain injury. *Brain Injury, 3*, 79–90.

Ellis, A. (1962). *Reason and emotion in psychotherapy*. New York: Lyle Stuart.

Ellis, D. W. (1989). Neuropsychotherapy. In D. Ellis & A. L. Christensen (Eds.), *Neuropsychological treatment after brain injury* (pp. 241–270). Boston: Kluver Academic Publishers.

Elsass, L., & Kinsella, G. (1987). Social interaction following severe closed head injury. *Psychological Medicine, 17*, 67–78.

Epperson-Sebour, M. M., & Rifkin, E. W. (1985). Center for living: Trauma aftercare and outcomes. *Maryland Medical Journal, 34*, 1187–1192.

Ethier, M., Baribeau, J., & Braun, C. (1989a). Computer dispensed cognitive perceptual training of closed head injury patients after spontaneous recovery. Study 1. Speeded tasks. *Canadian Journal of Rehabilitation, 3*, 7–16.

Ethier, M., Baribeau, J., & Braun, C. (1989b). Computer dispensed cognitive perceptual training of closed head injury patients after spontaneous recovery. Study 2. Unspeeded tasks. *Canadian Journal of Rehabilitation*, 2, 223–233.

Evans, C., & Skidmore, B. (1989). Rehabilitation in the community. In R. L. Wood & P. G. Eames (Eds.), *Models of brain injury rehabilitation* (pp. 59–74). London: Chapman & Hall.

Evans, R. W., Gualtieri, C. T., & Patterson, D. (1987). Treatment of chronic closed head injury with psychostimulant drugs: A controlled case study and an appropriate evaluation procedure. *Journal of Nervous and Mental Disease, 175*, 106–110.

Falloon, I. R., Boyd, J. L., & McGill, C. W. (1984). *Family care of schizophrenia*. New York: Guilford Press.

Fennell, M. (1989). Depression. In K. Hawton, P. M. Salkovskis, J. Kirk, & D. M. Clark (Eds.), *Cognitive behavior therapy for psychiatric problems: A practical guide* (pp. 169–234). Oxford: Oxford University Press.

Florian, V., Katz, S., & Lahav, V. (1991). Impact of traumatic brain damage on family dynamics and functioning: A review. *International Disability Studies, 13*, 150–157.

Folstein, M. F., Folstein, S. E., & McHugh, P. R. (1975). "Mini Mental State": A practical method for grading the cognitive state of patients for the clinician. *Journal of Psychiatric Research, 12,* 189–198.

Fordyce, D. J., & Roueche, J. R. (1986). Changes in perspectives of disability among patients, staff, and relatives during rehabilitation of brain injury. *Rehabilitation Psychology, 31,* 217–229.

Fordyce, D. J., Roueche, J. R., & Prigatano, G. P. (1983). Enhanced emotional reactions in chronic head trauma patients. *Journal of Neurology, Neurosurgery and Psychiatry, 46,* 620–624.

Forssmann-Falck, R., & Christian, F. M. (1989). The use of group therapy as a treatment modality for behavioral change following head injury. *Psychiatric Medicine, 7,* 43–50.

Fowler, R. S., Hart, J., & Sheehan, M. (1972). A prosthetic memory: An application of the prosthetic environment concept. *Rehabilitation Counselling Bulletin, 16,* 80–85.

Foxx, R. M., Marchand-Martella, N. E., Martella, R. C., Braunling-McMorrow, D. B., & McMorrow, M. J. (1988). Teaching a problem solving strategy to closed head injured adults. *Behavioral Residential Treatment, 3,* 193–210.

Foxx, R. M., Martella, R. C., & Marchand-Martella, N. E. (1989). The acquisition, maintenance, and generalization of problem solving skills by closed head injured adults. *Behavior Therapy, 20,* 61–76.

Frankowski, R. F. (1986). Descriptive epidemiologic studies of head injury in the United States: 1974–1984. *Advances in Psychosomatic Medicine, 16,* 153–172.

Freeman, M. R., Mittenberg, W., Dicowden, M., & Bat-Ami, M. (1992). Executive and compensatory memory retraining in traumatic brain injury. *Brain Injury, 6,* 65–70.

Fryer, L. J., & Haffey, W. J. (1987). Cognitive rehabilitation and community readaptation: Outcomes from two program models. *Journal of Head Trauma Rehabilitation, 2,* 51–63.

Gajar, A., Schloss, P. J., Schloss, C. N., & Thompson, C. K. (1984). Effects of feedback and self monitoring on head trauma youth's conversation skills. *Journal of Applied Behavior Analysis, 17,* 353–358.

Geva, N., & Stern, J. M. (1985). The use of dreams as a psychotherapeutic technique with brain injured patients. *Scandinavian Journal of Rehabilitation Medicine, Suppl. 12,* 47–49.

Giles, G. M., & Clark-Wilson, J. (1988a). Functional skills in severe brain injury. In I. Fussey & G. M. Giles (Eds.), *Rehabilitation of the severely brain injured adult: A practical approach* (pp. 69–101). London: Croom Helm.

Giles, G. M., & Clark-Wilson, J. (1988b). The use of behavioral techniques in functional skills training after severe brain injury. *American Journal of Occupational Therapy, 42,* 658–665.

Giles, G. M., & Fussey, I. (1988). Models of brain injury rehabilitation: From theory to practice. In I. Fussey & G. M. Giles (Eds.), *Rehabilitation of the severely brain injured adult: A practical approach* (pp. 1–30). London: Croom Helm.

Giles, G. M., Fussey, I., & Burgess, P. (1988). The behavioral treatment of verbal interaction skills following severe head injury: A single case study. *Brain Injury, 2,* 75–79.

Giles, G. M., & Shore, M. (1989). A rapid method for teaching severely brain injured adults how to wash and dress. *Archives of Physical and Medical Rehabilitation, 70,* 156–158.

Glasser, W. (1965). *Reality therapy.* New York: Harper & Row.

Glassman, L. R. (1991). Music therapy and bibliotherapy in the rehabilitation of traumatic brain injury: A case study. *The Arts in Psychotherapy, 18,* 149–156.

Gloag, D. (1985). Rehabilitation after head injury 2: Behavior and emotional problems, long term needs, and the requirements for services. *British Medical Journal, 290,* 913–916.

Glosser, G., & Deser, T. (1990). Patterns of discourse production among neurological patients with fluent language disorders. *Brain and Language, 40,* 67–88.

Gobble, E. M., Henry, K., Pfahl, K., & Smith, G. J. (1987). Work adjustment services. In M. Ylvisaker & E. M. Gobble (Eds.), *Community re-entry for head injured adults* (pp. 221–258). San Diego, CA: College Hill Press.

Gobiet, G. (1989). Improved clinical outcome with early rehabilitation. *Neurosurgical Review, 12*(Suppl. 1), 143–146.

Godfrey, H. P. D., Bishara, S. N., Partridge, F. M., & Knight, R. G. (1993a). Neuropsychological impairment and return to work following closed head injury: Implications for clinical management. *New Zealand Medical Journal, 106*, 301–303.

Godfrey, H. P. D., & Knight, R. G. (1985). Cognitive rehabilitation of memory functioning in dysmnesic alcoholics. *Journal of Consulting and Clinical Psychology, 53*, 555–557.

Godfrey, H. P. D., & Knight, R. G. (1987). Interventions for amnesics: A review. *British Journal of Clinical Psychology, 26*, 83–91.

Godfrey H. P. D., & Knight, R. G. (1988). Memory training and behavioral rehabilitation of a severely head injured adult. *Archives of Physical and Medical Rehabilitation, 69*, 458–460.

Godfrey, H. P. D., Knight, R. G., & Bishara, S. N. (1991). The relationship between social skill and family problem solving following very severe closed head injury. *Brain Injury, 5*, 207–211.

Godfrey, H. P. D., Knight, R. G., Marsh, N. V., Moroney, B., & Bishara, S. N. (1989). Social interaction and speed of information processing following very severe head injury. *Psychological Medicine, 19*, 175–182.

Godfrey, H. P. D., Knight, R. G., & Partridge, F. M. (1994). Emotional adjustment following closed head injury: A stress-appraisal-coping formulation. Unpublished manuscript. Dunedin, New Zealand: University of Otago, Clinical Psychology Research and Training Center.

Godfrey, H. P. D., Partridge, F. M., Knight, R. G., & Bishara, S. N. (1993b). Course of insight disorder and emotional dysfunction following closed head injury: A controlled cross-sectional follow-up study. *Journal of Clinical and Experimental Neuropsychology, 15*, 503–515.

Godfrey, H. P. D., & Smith, L. M. (1992). Psychosocial outcome of closed head injury: Nature, assessment and management. Unpublished manuscript. Dunedin, New Zealand: University of Otago, Department of Psychology.

Goldstein, F. C., & Levin, H. S. (1987). Disorders of reasoning and problem solving ability. In M. J. Meier, A. L. Benton, & L. Diller (Eds.), *Neuropsychological rehabilitation* (pp. 327–354). New York: Churchill Livingstone.

Goldstein, F. C., & Levin, H. S. (1991). Question asking strategies after severe closed head injury. *Brain and Cognition, 17*, 23–30.

Goldstein, F. C., Levin, H. S., & Boake, C. (1989). Conceptual encoding following severe closed head injury. *Cortex, 25*, 541–554.

Goldstein, G., & Ruthven, L. (1983). *Rehabilitation of the brain damaged adult.* New York: Plenum Press.

Goldstein, K. (1952). The effect of brain damage on the personality. *Psychiatry, 15*, 245–260.

Goodman-Smith, A., & Turnbull, J. (1983). A behavioral approach to the rehabilitation of severely brain injured adults. *Physiotherapy, 69*, 393–396.

Gordon, W. A. (1987). Methodological considerations in cognitive rehabilitation. In M. J. Meier, A. L. Benton, & L. Diller (Eds.), *Neuropsychological rehabilitation* (pp. 71–111). New York: Churchill Livingstone.

Gordon, W. A., & Hibbard, M. R. (1992). Critical issues in cognitive rehabilitation. *Neuropsychology, 6*, 361–370.

Grafman, J. (1984). Memory assessment and remediation in brain injured patients: From theory to practice. In B. A. Edelstein & E. T. Couture (Eds.), *Behavioral assessment and rehabilitation of the traumatically brain damaged* (pp. 151–190). New York: Plenum Press.

Gray, J. M., & Robertson, I. (1989). Remediation of attentional difficulties following brain injury: Three experimental single case studies. *Brain Injury, 3*, 163–170.

Grinspun, D. R. (1987). Teaching families of traumatic brain injured adults. *Critical Care Nursing Quarterly, 10*, 61–72.

Gronwall, D. M. (1977). Paced Auditory Serial-Addition Task: A measure of recovery from concussion. *Perceptual and Motor Skills, 44*, 367–373.

Gross, Y., Ben-Nahum, Z., & Munk, G. (1982). Techniques and application of simultaneous information processing. In L. Trexler (Ed.), *Cognitive rehabilitation: Conceptualization and intervention* (pp. 223–239). New York: Plenum Press.

Gualtieri, C. T., & Evans, R. E. (1988). Stimulant treatment for the neurobehavioral sequelae of traumatic brain injury. *Brain Injury, 2*, 273–290.

Haffey, W. J., & Abrams, D. L. (1991). Employment outcomes for participants in a brain injury work reentry program: Preliminary findings. *Journal of Head Trauma Rehabilitation, 6*, 24–34.

Haffey, W. J., & Lewis, F. D. (1989). Programming for occupational outcomes following traumatic brain injury. *Rehabilitation Psychology, 34*, 147–158.

Haffey, W. J., & Scibak, J. W. (1989). Management of aggressive behavior following traumatic brain injury. In D. Ellis & A. L. Christensen (Eds.), *Neuropsychological treatment after brain injury* (pp. 317–362). Boston: Kluver Academic Publishers.

Hahleg, K., & Markman, H. J. (1988). Effectiveness of behavioral marital therapy: Empirical status of behavioral techniques in preventing and alleviating marital distress. *Journal of Consulting and Clinical Psychology, 56*, 440–447.

Halford, W. K., & Hayes, R. (1991). Psychosocial rehabilitation of chronic schizophrenic patients: Recent findings on social skills training and family psychoeducation. *Clinical Psychology Review, 11*, 23–44.

Hamilton, M. (1959). The assessment of anxiety states by rating. *British Journal of Medical Psychology, 32*, 50–55.

Harrington, D. E., & Levandowski, D. H. (1987). Efficacy of an educationally based cognitive retraining program for the traumatically head injured as measured by LNNB pre and post test scores. *Brain Injury, 1*, 65–72.

Haut, M. W., Petros, T. V., Frank, R. G., & Haut, J. S. (1991). Speed of information processing within semantic memory following severe closed head injury. *Brain and Cognition, 17*, 31–41.

Hawton, K., & Kirk, J. (1989). Problem solving. In K. Hawton, P. M. Salkovskis, J. Kirk, & D. M. Clark (Eds.), *Cognitive behavior therapy for psychiatric problems: A practical guide* (pp. 406–426). Oxford: Oxford University Press.

Hegel, M. T. (1988). Application of a token economy with a noncompliant closed head injured male. *Brain Injury, 2*, 333–338.

Hegeman, K. M. (1988). A care plan for the family of a brain trauma client. *Rehabilitation Nursing, 13*, 254–258.

Heilbronner, R. L., Roueche, S. A., Everson, S. A., & Epler, L. (1989). Comparing patient perspectives of disability and treatment effects with quality of participation in a post-acute brain injury rehabilitation program. *Brain Injury, 3*, 387–395.

Heilman, K. M., Safran, A., & Geschwin, N. (1971). Closed head trauma and aphasia. *Journal of Neurology, Neurosurgery and Psychiatry, 34*, 265–269.

Helffenstein, D. A., & Wechsler, F. S. (1982). The use of interpersonal process recall (IPR) in the remediation of interpersonal and communication skills deficits in the newly brain injured. *Clinical Neuropsychology, 4*, 139–143.

Hinkeldey, N. S., & Corrigan, J. D. (1990). The structure of head-injured patients' neurobehavioral complaints: A preliminary study. *Brain Injury, 4*, 115–133.

Hollon, T. H. (1973). Behavior modification in a community hospital rehabilitation unit. *Archives of Physical and Medical Rehabilitation, 54*, 65–68.

Horton, A. M., & Howe, N. R. (1981). Behavioral treatment of the traumatically brain injured: A case study. *Perceptual and Motor Skills, 53*, 349–350.

Howlin, P., & Rutter, M. (1989). *Treatment of autistic children*. Chichester: John Wiley.

Intagliata, J., Willer, B., & Egri, G. (1988). The role of the family in delivering case management services. In M. Harris & I. I. Bachrach (Eds.), *Clinical case management: New directions for mental health services*, No. 40 (pp. 39–50) San Francisco: Jossey-Bass.

Jackson, R. D., Corrigan, J. D., & Arnett, J. A. (1985). Amitriptyline for agitation in head injury. *Archives of Physical and Medical Rehabilitation, 66*, 180–181.

Jacobs, H. E. (1989). Long term family intervention. In D. Ellis & A. L. Christensen (Eds.), *Neuropsychological treatment after brain injury* (pp. 297–316). Boston: Kluver Academic Publishers.

Jacobson, N. S., & Margolin, G. (1979). *Marital therapy: Strategies based on social learning and behavior exchange principles*. New York: Brunner/Mazel.

Jellinek, H. M., & Harvey, R. F. (1982). Vocational/educational services in a medical rehabilitation facility: Outcomes in spinal cord and brain injured patients. *Archives of Physical and Medical Rehabilitation, 63*, 87–88.

Jennett, B., & Teasdale, G. (1981). *Management of head injuries*. Philadelphia: F. A. Davis.

Johnson, D. A., & Newton, A. (1987). Social adjustment and interaction after severe head injury: Rationale and bases for intervention. *British Journal of Clinical Psychology, 26*, 289–298.

Johnson, J. R., & Higgins, L. (1987). Integration of family dynamics into the rehabilitation of the brain injured patient. *Rehabilitation Nursing, 12*, 320–322.

Johnston, M. V. (1991). Outcomes of community re-entry programs for brain injury survivors. Part 2. Further investigations. *Brain Injury, 5*, 155–168.

Johnston, M. V., & Lewis, F. D. (1991). Outcomes of community re-entry programs for brain injury survivors. Part 1. Independent living and productive activities. *Brain Injury, 5*, 141–154.

Jones, E. E., Cumming, J. D., & Horowitz, M. J. (1988). Another look at the nonspecific hypothesis of therapeutic effectiveness. *Journal of Consulting and Clinical Psychology, 56*, 48–55.

Kafner, F. H., & Grimm, L. G. (1980). Managing clinical change: A process model of therapy. *Behavior Modification, 4*, 419–444.

Kalat, J. W. (1981). *Biological psychology*. Belmont, CA: Wadsworth Publishing.

Kinsella, G., Ford, B., & Moran, C. (1989). Survival of social relationships following head injury. *International Disability Studies, 11*, 9–14.

Kinsella, G., Moran, C., Ford, B., & Ponsford, J. (1988). Emotional disorder and its assessment within the severe head injured population. *Psychological Medicine, 18*, 57–63.

Kirn, T. F. (1987). Cognitive rehabilitation aims to improve or replace memory functions in survivors of head injury. *Journal of the American Medical Association, 257*, 2400–2402.

Klonoff, P. S., O'Brien, K. P., Prigatano, G. P., Chiapello, D. A., & Cunningham, M. (1989). Cognitive retraining after traumatic brain injury and its role in facilitating awareness. *Journal of Head Trauma Rehabilitation, 4*, 37–45.

Klonoff, P., & Prigatano, G. P. (1987). Reactions of family members and clinical intervention after traumatic brain injury. In M. Ylvisaker & E. M. Gobble (Eds.), *Community reentry for head injured adults* (pp. 381–402). San Diego, CA: College Hill Press.

Knight, R. G. (1992). *The neuropsychology of degenerative brain disorders*. Hillsdale, NJ: Lawrence Erlbaum Associates.

Knight, R. G., Waal-Manning, H. J., & Spears, G. F. (1983). Some norms and reliability data for the State–Trait Anxiety Inventory and Zung Self Rating Depression Scale. *British Journal of Clinical Psychology, 22*, 245–249.

Kreutzer, J. S., Conder, R., Wehman, P., & Morrison, C. (1991). Compensatory strategies for enhancing independent living and vocational outcome following traumatic brain injury. *Cognitive Rehabilitation, 7*, 30–35.

Kreutzer, J. S., Gordon, W. A., & Wehman, P. (1989). Cognitive remediation following traumatic brain injury. *Rehabilitation Psychology, 34*, 117–130 (cf. Diller, 1989).

Lal, S., Merbitz, C. P., & Grip, J. C. (1988). Modification of function in head injured patients with Sinemet. *Brain Injury, 2*, 225–233.

Langley, M. J., Lindsay, W. P., Lam, C. S., & Priddy, D. A. (1990). A comprehensive alcohol abuse treatment program for persons with traumatic brain injury. *Brain Injury, 4*, 77–86.

Lawson, M. J., & Rice, D. N. (1989). Effects of training in use of executive strategies on a verbal memory problem resulting from closed head injury. *Journal of Experimental and Clinical Psychology, 11*, 842–854.

Lazarus, R. S., & Folkman, S. (1984). *Stress appraisal and coping*. New York: Springer.

Letoff, S. (1983). Psychopathology in the light of brain injury: A case study. *Journal of Clinical Neuropsychology, 5*, 51–63.

Levin, H. S. (1990a). Cognitive rehabilitation: Unproven but promising. *Archives of Neurology, 47*, 223–224.

Levin, H. S. (1990b). Memory deficit after closed head injury. *Journal of Clinical and Experimental Neuropsychology, 12*, 129–153.

Levin, H. S., & Goldstein, F. C. (1986). Organization of verbal memory after severe closed-head injury. *Journal of Clinical and Experimental Neuropsychology, 8*, 643–656.

Levin, H. S., Goldstein, F. C., High, W. M., & Eisenberg, H. M. (1988). Disproportionately severe memory deficits in relation to normal intellectual functioning after closed head injury. *Journal of Neurology, Neurosurgery and Psychiatry, 51*, 14–20.

Lewin, W. (1968). Rehabilitation after head injury. *British Medical Journal, 24*, 465–470.

Lewinsohn, P. M., Munoz, R. F., Youngren, M. A., & Zeiss, A. M. (1986). *Control your depression*. New York: Prentice Hall.

Lewis, N. R. (1966). Rehabilitation after head injury. *Proceedings of the Royal Society of Medicine, 59*, 623–625.

Lezak, M. D. (1978). Living with the characterologically altered brain injured patient. *Journal of Clinical Psychiatry, 39*, 592–598.

Lezak, M. D. (1986). Psychological implications of traumatic brain damage for the patient's family. *Rehabilitation Psychology, 31*, 241–250.

Lezak, M. D. (1987). Relationships between personality disorders, social disturbances, and physical disability following traumatic brain injury. *Journal of Head Trauma Rehabilitation, 2*, 57–69.

Lezak, M. D. (1988). Brain damage is a family affair. *Journal of Clinical and Experimental Neuropsychology, 10*, 111–123.

Liles, B. Z., Coelho, C. A., Duffy, R. J., & Zalagens, M. R. (1989). Effects of elicitation procedures on the narratives of normal and closed head-injured adults. *Journal of Speech and Hearing Disorders, 54*, 356–366.

Linscott, R. J., Knight, R. G., & Godfrey, H. P. D. (1993). Manual for the profile of functional impairment in communication (PFIC). Unpublished manuscript. Dunedin, New Zealand: University of Otago, Department of Psychology.

Lipper, S., & Tuchman, M. M. (1976). Treatment of chronic post traumatic organic brain syndrome with dextroamphetamine: First reported case. *Journal of Nervous and Mental Disease, 162*, 366–371.

Lira, F. T., Carne, W., & Masri, A. M. (1983). Treatment of anger and impulsivity in a brain damaged patient: A case study applying stress inoculation. *International Journal of Clinical Neuropsychology, 5*, 159–160.

Liss, M., & Willer, B. (1990). Traumatic brain injury and marital relationships: A literature review. *International Journal of Rehabilitation Research, 13*, 309–320.

Livingston, M. G., Brooks, D. N., & Bond, M. R. (1985a). Patient outcome in the year following severe head injury and relatives' psychiatric and social functioning. *Journal of Neurology, Neurosurgery and Psychiatry, 48*, 876–881.

Livingston, M. G., Brooks, D. N., & Bond, M. R. (1985b). Three months after severe head injury: Psychiatric and social impact on relatives. *Journal of Neurology, Neurosurgery and Psychiatry, 48*, 870–875.

Lyons, J. L., & Morse, A. R. (1988). A therapeutic work program for head injured adults. *American Journal of Occupational Therapy, 42*, 364–370.

Lysaght, R., & Bodenhamer, E. (1990). The use of relaxation training to enhance functional outcomes in adults with traumatic head injuries. *American Journal of Occupational Therapy, 44*, 797–802.

MacKay, L. E., Bernstein, B. A., Chapman, P. E., Morgan, A. S., & Milazzo, L. S. (1992). Early intervention in severe head injury: Long term benefits of a formalized program. *Archives of Physical Medicine and Rehabilitation, 73*, 635–641.

Malec, J. (1984). Training the brain injured client in behavioral self management skills. In B. A. Edelstein & E. T. Couture (Eds.), *Behavioral assessment and rehabilitation of the traumatically brain damaged* (pp. 121–150). New York: Plenum Press.

Malkmus, D. D. (1989). Community re-entry: Cognitive–communication intervention within a social skill context. *Topics in Language Disorders, 9*, 50–66.

Mandelberg, I. A., & Brooks, D. N. (1975). Cognitive recovery after severe head injury. 1. Serial testing on the Wechsler Adult Intelligence Scale. *Journal of Neurology, Neurosurgery and Psychiatry, 38*, 1121–1126.

Marlatt, G. A., & Gordon, J. R. (1985). *Relapse prevention: Maintenance strategies in the treatment of addictive behaviors*. New York: Guilford Press.

Marquardt, T. P., Stoll, J., & Sussman, H. (1988). Disorders of communication in acquired cerebral trauma. *Journal of Learning Disabilities, 21*, 340–351.

Marsh, N. V., Knight, R. G., & Godfrey, H. P. D. (1990). Long-term psychosocial adjustment following very severe closed head injury. *Neuropsychology, 4*, 13–27.

Mauss-Clum, N., & Ryan, M. (1981). Brain injury and the family. *Journal of Neurosurgical Nursing, 13*, 165–169.

McAllister, T. W. (1985). Carbamazepine in mixed frontal lobe and psychiatric disorders. *Journal of Clinical Psychiatry, 46*, 393–394.

McClelland, R. J. (1988). Psychosocial sequelae of head injury, anatomy of a relationship. *British Journal of Psychiatry, 153*, 141–146.

McGlynn, S. M. (1990). Behavioral approaches to neuropsychological rehabilitation. *Psychological Bulletin, 108*, 420–441.

McGlynn, S. M., & Schacter, D. L. (1990). Unawareness of deficits in neuropsychological syndromes. *Journal of Clinical and Experimental Neuropsychology, 11*, 143–205.

McKinlay, W. W., & Brooks, D. N. (1984). Methodological problems in assessing psychosocial recovery following severe head injury. *Journal of Clinical Neuropsychology, 6*, 87–99.

McKinlay, W. W., Brooks, D. N., Bond, M. R., Martinage, D. P., & Marshall, M. M. (1981). The short-term outcome of severe blunt head injury as reported by relatives of the injured persons. *Journal of Neurology, Neurosurgery and Psychiatry, 44*, 527–533.

McKinlay, W. W., & Hickox, A. (1988). How can families help in the rehabilitation of the head injured? *Journal of Head Trauma Rehabilitation, 3*, 64–72.

McMordie, W. R., Rogers, K. F., & Barker, S. L. (1991). Consumer satisfaction with services provided to head injured patients and their families. *Brain Injury, 5*, 43–51.

Meichenbaum, D. (1977). *Cognitive behavior modification: An integrative approach*. New York: Plenum Press.

Meichenbaum, D. H., & Goodman, J. (1971). Training impulsive children to talk to themselves: A means of developing self-control. *Journal of Abnormal Psychology, 77*, 115–126.

Meier, M. J., Strauman, S., & Thompson, W. G. (1987). Individual differences in neuropsychological recovery: An overview. In M. J. Meier, A. L. Benton, & L. Diller (Eds.), *Neuropsychological rehabilitation* (pp. 71–111). New York: Churchill Livingstone.

Mentis, M., & Prutting, C. A. (1987). Cohesion in the discourse of normal and head injured adults. *Journal of Speech and Hearing Research, 30*, 88–98.

Middleton, D. K., Lambert, M. J., & Seggar, L. B. (1991). Neuropsychological rehabilitation: Microcomputer assisted treatment of brain injured adults. *Perceptual and Motor Skills, 72*, 527–530.

Mills, V. M., Nesbeda, T., Katz, D. I., & Alexander, M. P. (1992). Outcomes for traumatically brain injured patients following post acute rehabilitation programs. *Brain Injury, 6*, 219–228.

Minium, E. W. (1970). *Statistical reasoning in psychology and education.* New York: John Wiley.

Molloy, M. (1983). New perspectives in cognitive rehabilitation. *Australian Rehabilitation Review, 7*, 34–37.

Moore, A. D., Stambrook, M., & Peters, L. C. (1989). Coping strategies and adjustment after closed-head injury: A cluster analytical approach. *Brain Injury, 3*, 171–175.

Morris, J., & Bleiberg, J. (1986). Neuropsychological rehabilitation and traditional psychotherapy. *International Journal of Clinical Neuropsychology, 8*, 133–135.

Muir, C. A., & Haffey, W. J. (1984). Psychological and neuropsychological interventions in the mobile mourning process. In B. A. Edelstein & E. T. Couture (Eds.), *Behavioral assessment and rehabilitation of the traumatically brain damaged* (pp. 247–272). New York: Plenum Press.

Mysiw, W. J., & Jackson, R. D. (1987). Tricyclic antidepressant therapy after traumatic brain injury. *Journal of Head Trauma Rehabilitation, 2*, 34–42.

Mysiw, W. J., Jackson, R. D., & Corrigan, J. D. (1988). Amitriptyline for post traumatic agitation. *American Journal of Physical Medicine and Rehabilitation, 67*, 29–33.

Najenson, T., Groswasser, Z., Mendelson, L., & Hackett, P. (1980). Rehabilitation outcome of brain damaged patients after severe head injury. *International Rehabilitation Medicine, 2*, 17–22.

Namerow, N. S. (1987). Cognitive and behavioral aspects of brain-injury rehabilitation. *Neurologic Clinics, 5*, 569–583.

Nelson, H. E. (1982). *National Adult Reading Test (NART) for the assessment of premorbid intelligence in patients with dementia: Test manual.* Windsor: NFER-Nelson Publishing Co.

Nelson, H. E., & O'Connell, A. (1978). Dementia: The estimation of premorbid intelligence levels using the New Adult Reading Test. *Cortex, 14*, 234–244.

Niemann, H., Ruff, R. M., & Baser, C. A. (1990). Computer assisted attention retraining in head injured individuals: A controlled efficacy study of an outpatient program. *Journal of Consulting and Clinical Psychology, 58*, 811–817.

Novack, T. A., & Richards, J. S. (1991). Coping with denial among family members. *Archives of Physical and Medical Rehabilitation, 72*, 521.

O'Connor, M., & Cermack, L. S. (1987). Rehabilitation of organic memory disorders. In M. J. Meier, A. L. Benton, & L. Diller (Eds.), *Neuropsychological rehabilitation* (pp. 260–280). New York: Churchill Livingstone.

Oddy, M., Coughlan, T., Tyerman, A., & Jenkins, D. (1985). Social adjustment after closed head injury: A further follow-up seven years after injury. *Journal of Neurology, Neurosurgery and Psychiatry, 48*, 564–568.

Oddy, M., & Humphrey, M. (1980). Social recovery during the year following severe head injury. *Journal of Neurology, Neurosurgery and Psychiatry, 43*, 798–802.

Oddy, M., Humphrey, M., & Uttley, D. (1978a). Stresses upon the relatives of head injured patients. *British Journal of Psychiatry, 133*, 507–513.

Oddy, M., Humphrey, M., & Uttley, D. (1978b). Subjective impairment and social recovery after closed head injury. *Journal of Neurology, 41*, 611–616.

O'Shanick, G. J. (1988). Psychotropic management of behavioral disorders after head trauma. *Psychiatric Medicine, 6*, 67–82.

O'Shanick, G. J. (1989). Behavior change following head injury: Clinical assessment and intervention. *Psychiatric Medicine, 7*, 1–10.

Paniak, C. E., Shore, D. L., & Rourke, B. P. (1989). Recovery of memory after severe closed-head injury: Dissociations in recovery of memory as predictors of outcome. *Journal of Clinical and Experimental Neuropsychology, 11*, 631–644.

Panting, A., & Merry, P. H. (1972). The long term rehabilitation of severe head injuries with particular reference to the need for social and medical support for the patient's family. *Rehabilitation, 82*, 33–37.

Partridge, F. M. (1991). Adjustment following severe closed head injury. Unpublished doctoral dissertation. Dunedin, New Zealand: University of Otago.

Perry, J. (1983). Rehabilitation of the neurologically disabled patient: Principles, practice, and scientific basis. *Journal of Neurosurgery, 58*, 799–816.

Peters, L. C., Stambrook, M., Moore, A. D., & Esses, L. (1990). Psychosocial sequelae of closed head injury: Effects on marital relationship. *Brain Injury, 4*, 39–47.

Peters, L. C., Stambrook, M., Moore, A. D., Zubek, E., Dubo, H., & Blumenschein, S. (1992). Differential effects of spinal cord injury and head injury on marital adjustment. *Brain Injury, 6*, 461–467.

Peters, M. D., Gluck, M., & McCormick, M. (1992). Behavior rehabilitation of the challenging client in less restrictive settings. *Brain, 16*, 299–314.

Piasetsky, E. B., Ben-Yishay, Y., Weinberg, J., & Diller, L. (1982). The systematic remediation of specific disorders: Selected application of methods derived in a clinical research setting. In L. Trexler (Ed.), *Cognitive rehabilitation: Conceptualization and intervention* (pp. 205–223). New York: Plenum Press.

Ponsford, J. L., & Kinsella, G. (1988). Evaluation of a remedial program for attentional deficits following closed head injury. *Journal of Clinical and Experimental Neuropsychology, 10*, 693–708.

Ponsford, J., & Kinsella, G. (1992). Attentional deficits following closed head injury. *Journal of Clinical and Experimental Neuropsychology, 14*, 828–838.

Prickel, D., & McLean, B. (1989). Vocational rehabilitation of the head injured person in the rural setting. *Cognitive Rehabilitation*, November–December, 22–26.

Prigatano, G. P. (1986). Personality and psychosocial consequences of brain injury. In G. P. Prigatano (Ed.), *Neuropsychological rehabilitation after brain injury* (pp. 29–49). Baltimore: Johns Hopkins University Press.

Prigatano, G. P. (1987a). Personality and psychosocial consequences after brain injury. In M. J. Meier, A. L. Benton, & L. Diller (Eds.), *Neuropsychological rehabilitation* (pp. 355–379). New York: Churchill Livingstone.

Prigatano, G. P. (1987b). Recovery and cognitive retraining after craniocerebral trauma. *Journal of Learning Disabilities, 20*, 603–613.

Prigatano, G. P. (1992). Personality disturbances associated with traumatic brain injury. *Journal of Consulting and Clinical Psychology, 60*, 360–368.

Prigatano, G. P., & Fordyce, D. J. (1986a). Cognitive dysfunction and psychosocial adjustment after brain injury. In G. P. Prigatano (Ed.), *Neuropsychological rehabilitation after brain injury* (pp. 1–16). Baltimore: Johns Hopkins University Press.

Prigatano, G. P., & Fordyce, D. J. (1986b). The neuropsychological rehabilitation program at Presbyterian Hospital, Oklahoma City. In G. P. Prigatano (Ed.), *Neuropsychological rehabilitation after brain injury* (pp. 96–118). Baltimore: Johns Hopkins University Press.

Prigatano, G. P., Fordyce, D. J., Zeiner, H. K., Roueche, J. R., Pepping, M., & Wood, B. C. (1984). Neuropsychological rehabilitation after closed head injury in young adults. *Journal of Neurology, Neurosurgery and Psychiatry, 47*, 505–513.

Prigatano, G. P., Fordyce, D. J., Zeiner, H. K., Roueche, J. R., Pepping, M., & Wood, B. C. (1986a). The outcome of neuropsychological rehabilitation efforts. In G. P. Prigatano (Ed.), *Neuropsychological rehabilitation after brain injury* (pp. 119–132). Baltimore: Johns Hopkins University Press.

Prigatano, G. P., Roueche, J. R., & Fordyce, D. J. (1986b). Nonaphasic language disturbances after brain injury. In G. P. Prigatano (Ed.), *Neuropsychological rehabilitation after brain injury* (pp. 18–27). Baltimore: Johns Hopkins University Press.

Quine, S., Pierce, J. P., & Lyle, D. M. (1988). Relatives as lay therapists for the severely head injured. *Brain Injury, 2,* 139–149.

Rankin, H. (1982). Control rather than abstinence as a goal in the treatment of excessive gambling. *Behavior Research and Therapy, 20,* 185–187.

Ranseen, J. D. (1985). Comprehensive rehabilitation of head injured adults. *Maryland Medical Journal, 34,* 1176–1182.

Rao, N., Rosenthal, M., Cronin-Stubbs, D., Lambert, R., Barnes, P., & Swanson, B. (1990). Return to work after rehabilitation following traumatic brain injury. *Brain Injury, 4,* 49–56.

Rao, N., Sulton, L., Young, C. L., & Harvey, R. F. (1986). Rehabilitation team and family assessment of the initial home pass. *Archives of Physical and Medical Rehabilitation, 67,* 759–761.

Rattok, J., Ben-Yishay, Y., Ezrachi, O., Lakin, P., Piasetsky, E., Ross, B., Silver, S., Vakil, E., Zide, E., & Diller, L. (1992). Outcome of different treatment mixes in a multidimensional neuropsychological rehabilitation program. *Neuropsychology, 6,* 395–416.

Reinvang, I. (1987). Neuropsychological rehabilitation in Norway and Sweden. In M. J. Meier, A. L. Benton, & L. Diller (Eds.), *Neuropsychological rehabilitation* (pp. 423–429). New York: Churchill Livingstone.

Rey, A. (1964). L'examen psychologique dans les cas d'encephalopathie traumatique. *Archives de Psychologie, 28,* 286–340.

Richardson, J. E. (1990). *Clinical and neuropsychological aspects of closed head injury.* London: Taylor & Francis.

Ridley, B. (1989). Family response in head injury: Denial or hope for the future. *Social Science and Medicine, 29,* 555–561.

Robertson, I., Gray, J., & McKenzie, S. (1988). Microcomputer-based cognitive rehabilitation of visual neglect: Three multiple baseline single case studies. *Brain Injury, 2,* 151–163.

Robinson, E. (1960). *Effective study.* New York: Harper & Row.

Rogers, P. M., & Kreutzer, J. S. (1984). Family crises following head injury: A network intervention strategy. *Journal of Neurosurgical Nursing, 16,* 343–346.

Rose, M. (1988). Medical considerations in brain injury rehabilitation. In I. Fussey & G. M. Giles (Eds.), *Rehabilitation of the severely brain injured adult: A practical approach* (pp. 30–43). London: Croom Helm.

Rosenbaum, M., & Najenson, T. (1976). Changes in life patterns and symptoms of low mood as reported by wives of severely brain-injured soldiers. *Journal of Consulting and Clinical Psychology, 44,* 881–888.

Rosenberg, M. (1965). *Society and the adolescent self-image.* Princeton, NJ: Princeton University Press.

Rosenthal, M. (1984). Strategies for intervention with families of brain injured patients. In B. A. Edelstein & E. T. Couture (Eds.), *Behavioral assessment and rehabilitation of the traumatically brain damaged* (pp. 227–246). New York: Plenum Press.

Rosenthal, M. (1989). Response to "Psychotherapeutic interventions with traumatically brain-injured patients." *Rehabilitation Psychology, 34,* 115–116 (cf. Cicerone, 1989).

Ruff, R. M., Baser, C. A., Johnston, J. W., Marshall, L. J., Klauber, S. K., Klauber, M. R., & Minteer, M. (1989). Neuropsychological rehabilitation: An experimental study with head injured patients. *Journal of Head Trauma Rehabilitation, 4,* 20–36.

Russell, E. W. (1975). A multiple scoring method for the assessment of complex memory functions. *Journal of Consulting and Clinical Psychology, 43,* 800–809.

Russell, W. R. (1932). Cerebral involvement in head injury: A study based on the examination of 200 cases. *Brain, 55,* 549–602.

Russell, W. R. (1971). *The traumatic amnesias.* Oxford: Oxford University Press.

Sahgal, V., & Heinemann, A. (1989). Recovery of function during inpatient rehabilitation for moderate traumatic brain injury. *Scandinavian Journal of Rehabilitation Medicine, 21,* 71–79.

Sanders, M. R. (1992). New directions in behavioral family intervention with children: From clinical management to prevention. *New Zealand Journal of Psychology, 21*, 25–36.

Sanguinetti, M., & Catanzaro, M. (1987). A comparison of discharge teaching on the consequences of brain injury. *Journal of Neuroscience Nursing, 19*, 271–275.

Sarno, M. T. (1980). The nature of verbal impairment after closed head injury. *Journal of Nervous and Mental Disease, 168*, 685–692.

Sarno, M. T. (1988). Head injury: Language and speech defects. *Scandinavian Journal of Rehabilitation Medicine, Suppl. 17*, 55–64.

Scherzer, B. P. (1986). Rehabilitation following severe head trauma: Results of a three-year program. *Archives of Physical Medicine and Rehabilitation, 67*, 366–373.

Schloss, P. J., Thompson, C. K., Gajar, A. H., & Schloss, C. N. (1985). Influence of self-monitoring on heterosexual conversational behaviors of head trauma youth. *Applied Research in Mental Retardation, 6*, 269–282.

Schmaling, K. B., Fruzzetti, A. E., & Jacobsen, N. (1989). Marital problems. In K. Hawton, P. M. Salkovskis, J. Kirk, & D. M. Clark (Eds.), *Cognitive behavior therapy for psychiatric problems: A practical guide* (pp. 339–369). Oxford: Oxford University Press.

Schmitter-Edgecombe, M., Marks, W., & Fahy, J. F. (1993). Semantic priming after closed head trauma: Automatic and attentional processes. *Neuropsychology, 7*, 136–148.

Schmitter-Edgecombe, M., Marks, W., Fahy, J. F., & Long, C. J. (1992). Effects of severe closed head injury on three stages of information processing. *Journal of Clinical and Experimental Neuropsychology, 14*, 717–737.

Series, C. (1992). The long term needs of people with head injury: A role for the community occupational therapist? *British Journal of Occupational Therapy, 55*, 94–98.

Shaffer, D., Garland, A., Gould, M., Gisher, P., & Trautman, P. (1988). Preventing teenage suicide: A critical review. *Journal of the American Academy of Child and Adolescent Psychiatry, 27*, 689–695.

Shaw, L. R., & McMahon, B. T. (1990). Family–staff conflict in the rehabilitation setting: Causes, consequences, and implications. *Brain Injury, 4*, 87–93.

Sherr, R. L., & Langenbahn, D. M. (1992). An approach to large scale outpatient neuropsychological rehabilitation. *Neuropsychology, 6*, 417–426.

Shum, D. H., McFarland, K., Bain, J. D., & Humphreys, M. S. (1990). Effects of closed head injury on attentional processes: An information processing stage analysis. *Journal of Clinical and Experimental Neuropsychology, 12*, 247–264.

Simon, K. B. (1988). Outpatient treatment for an adult with traumatic brain injury. *American Journal of Occupational Therapy, 42*, 247–251.

Slagle, D. A. (1990). Psychiatric disorders following closed head injury: An overview of biopsychological factors in their etiology and management. *International Journal of Psychiatry in Medicine, 20*, 1–35.

Smith, R. K. (1983). Prevocational programming in the rehabilitation of the head injured patient. *Physical Therapy, 63*, 2026–2029.

Soderstrom, S., Fogelsjoo, A., & Fugl-Meyer, K. S. (1988). A program for crisis intervention after traumatic brain injury. *Scandinavian Journal of Rehabilitation Medicine, Suppl. 17*, 47–49.

Sohlberg, M. M., & Mateer, C. A. (1987). Effectiveness of an attention training program. *Journal of Clinical and Experimental Neuropsychology, 9*, 117–130.

Sohlberg, M. M., & Mateer, C. (1989). Training use of compensatory memory books: A three stage behavioral approach. *Journal of Clinical and Experimental Neuropsychology, 11*, 871–891.

Sohlberg, M., White, O., Evans, E., & Mateer, C. (1992). Background and initial case studies into effects of prospective memory training. *Brain Injury, 6*, 129–138.

Spence, S. E., Godfrey, H. P. D., Bishara, S. N., & Knight, R. G. (1993). First impressions count: A controlled investigation of social skill following closed head injury. *British Journal of Clinical Psychology, 32*, 309–318.

Spielberger, C. D., Gorsuch, R. L., Lushene, R., Vagg, P. R., & Jacobs, G. A. (1983). *Manual for the State–Trait Anxiety Inventory: STAI (Form Y)*. Palo Alto, CA: Consulting Psychologists Press.

Spivack, G., Spettell, C. M., Ellis, D. W., & Ross, S. E. (1992). Effects of intensity of treatment and length of stay on rehabilitation outcomes. *Brain Injury, 6*, 419–434.

Stambrook, M., Moore, A. D., Peters, L. C., Deviaene, C., & Hawryluk, G. A. (1990). Effects of mild, moderate, and severe closed head injury on long term vocational status. *Brain Injury, 4*, 183–190.

Stern, B., & Stern, J. M. (1985). On the use of dreams as a means of diagnosis of brain injured patients. *Scandinavian Journal of Rehabilitation Medicine, Suppl. 12*, 44–46.

Stern, J. M. (1985). The quality of the psychotherapeutic process in brain injured patients. *Scandinavian Journal of Rehabilitation Medicine, Suppl. 12*, 42–43.

Stern, J. M., Groswasser, Z., Geva, N., Alis, R., Hochberg, J., Stern, B., & Yardeni, Y. (1985). Day center experience in rehabilitation of craniocerebral injured patients. *Scandinavian Journal of Rehabilitation Medicine, Suppl. 12*, 53–58.

Stern, J. M., & Stern, B. (1989). Visual imagery as a cognitive means of compensation for brain injury. *Brain Injury, 3*, 413–419.

Stuss, D. T., & Benson, D. F. (1984). Neuropsychological studies of the frontal lobes. *Psychological Bulletin, 95*, 3–28.

Stuss, D. T., & Gow, C. A. (1992). Frontal dysfunction after traumatic brain injury. *Neuropsychiatry, Neuropsychology and Behavioural Neurology, 5*, 272–282.

Symonds, C. (1962). Concussion and its sequelae. *Lancet, 1*, 1–5.

Szekeres, S. F., Ylvisaker, M., & Cohen, S. B. (1987). A framework for cognitive rehabilitation therapy. In M. Ylvisaker & E. M. Gobble (Eds.), *Community re-entry for head injured adults* (pp. 87–136). San Diego, CA: College Hill Press.

Tadir, M., & Stern, J. M. (1985). The mourning process with brain injured patients. *Scandinavian Journal of Rehabilitation Medicine, Suppl. 12*, 50–52.

Tate, R. L. (1987a). Behavior management techniques for organic psychosocial deficit incurred by severe head injury. *Scandinavian Journal of Rehabilitation Medicine, 19*, 19–24.

Tate, R. L. (1987b). Issues in the management of behavior disturbance as a consequence of severe head injury. *Scandinavian Journal of Rehabilitation Medicine, 19*, 13–18.

Tate, R. L., Fenelon, B., Manning, M. L., & Hunter, M. (1991). Patterns of neuropsychological impairment after severe blunt head injury. *Journal of Nervous and Mental Disease, 179*, 117–126.

Tate, R. L., Lulham, J. M., Broe, G. A., Strettles, B., & Pfaff, A. (1989). Psychosocial outcome for the survivors of severe blunt head injury: The results from a consecutive series of 100 patients. *Journal of Neurology, Neurosurgery and Psychiatry, 52*, 1128–1134.

Thomsen, I. V. (1974). The patient with severe head injury and his family: A follow-up study of 50 patients. *Scandinavian Journal of Rehabilitation Medicine, 61*, 180–183.

Thomsen, I. V. (1984). Late outcome of very severe blunt head trauma: A 10–15 year second follow-up. *Journal of Neurology, Neurosurgery and Psychiatry, 47*, 260–268.

Thomsen, I. V. (1987). Late psychosocial outcome in severe blunt head trauma. *Brain Injury, 1*, 131–143.

Trexler, L. E. (1987). Neuropsychological rehabilitation in the United States. In M. J. Meier, A. L. Benton, & L. Diller (Eds.), *Neuropsychological rehabilitation* (pp. 437–460). New York: Churchill Livingstone.

Turner, J. M., Green, G., & Braunling-McMorrow, D. (1990). Differential reinforcement of low rates of responding (DRL) to reduce dysfunctional social behaviors of a head injured man. *Behavioral Residential Treatment, 51*, 15–27.

Tyerman, A., & Humphrey, M. (1984). Changes in self-concept following severe head injury. *International Journal of Rehabilitation Research, 7*, 11–23.

Uomoto, J. M., & McLean, A. (1989). Care continuum in traumatic brain injury rehabilitation. *Rehabilitation Psychology, 34*, 71–79.

Vakil, E., Arbell, N., Gozlan, M., Hoofien, D., & Blachstein, H. (1992). Relative importance of informational units and their role in long-term recall by closed-head-injured patients and control groups. *Journal of Consulting and Clinical Psychology,* 60, 802–803.

Van Zomeren, A. H., Brouwer, W. H., & Deelman, B. G. (1984). Attentional deficits: The riddles of selectivity, speed, and alertness. In N. Brooks (Ed.), *Closed head injury: Psychological, social and family consequences.* Oxford: Oxford University Press.

Van Zomeren, A. H., & Deelman, B. G. (1976). Differential effects of simple and choice reaction after closed head injury. *Clinical Neurology and Neurosurgery, 79,* 81–90.

Vilkki, J. (1992). Cognitive flexibility and mental programming after closed head injuries and anterior or posterior cerebral excisions. *Neuropsychologia, 30,* 807–814.

Volpe, B. T., & McDowell, F. H. (1990). The efficacy of cognitive rehabilitation in patients with traumatic brain injury. *Archives of Neurology, 47,* 220–222.

Wagner, M. T., Williams, J. M., & Long, C. J. (1990). The role of social networks in recovery from head trauma. *International Journal of Clinical Neuropsychology, 12,* 131–137.

Walker, A. E. (1972). Summary for the international symposium on rehabilitation in head injury. *Scandinavian Journal of Rehabilitation Medicine, 4,* 145–146.

Webster, J. S., & Scott, R. R. (1983). The effects of self instructional training on attentional deficits following head injury. *International Journal of Clinical Neuropsychology, 5,* 69–74.

Webster-Stratton, C. (1989). Systematic comparison of consumer satisfaction of three cost effective parent training programs for conduct problem children. *Behavior Therapy, 20,* 103–115.

Weddell, R., Oddy, M., & Jenkins, D. (1980). Social adjustment after rehabilitation: A two year follow-up of patients with severe head injury. *Psychological Medicine, 10,* 257–263.

Wehman, P., Kreutzer, J. S., Stonnington, H. H., & Wood, W. (1988). Supported employment for persons with traumatic brain injury: A preliminary report. *Journal of Head Trauma Rehabilitation, 3,* 82–93.

Wehman, P., Kreutzer, J., West, M., Sherron, P., Diambra, J., Fry, R., Groah, C., Sale, P., & Killam, S. (1989a). Employment outcomes of persons following traumatic brain injury: Pre-injury, post injury, and supported employment. *Brain Injury, 3,* 397–412.

Wehman, P., Kreutzer, J., Wood, W., Stonnington, H., Diambra, J., & Morton, M. V. (1989b). Helping traumatically brain injured patients return to work with supported employment: Three case studies. *Archives of Physical and Medical Rehabilitation, 70,* 109–113.

Wehman, P., West, M., Fry, R., Sherron, P., Groah, C., Kreutzer, J., & Sale, P. (1989c). Effect of supported employment on the vocational outcomes of persons with traumatic brain injury. *Journal of Applied Behavior Analysis, 22,* 395–405.

Weinberg, R. M., Auerbach, S. H., & Moore, S. (1987). Pharmacologic treatment of cognitive deficits: A case study. *Brain Injury, 1,* 57–59.

Weiner, B., Heckhausen, H., & Meyer, W. U. (1972). Causal ascriptions and achievement behavior: A conceptual analysis of effort and reanalysis of locus of control. *Journal of Personality and Social Psychology, 21,* 239–248.

Wesoloski, M. D., & Zencius, A. H. (1994). *A practical guide to head injury rehabilitation: A focus on postacute residential rehabilitation.* New York: Plenum Press.

West, M., Wehman, P., Kregel, J., Kreutzer, J., Sherron, P., & Zasler, N. (1991). Costs of operating a supported work program for traumatically brain injured individuals. *Archives of Physical and Medical Rehabilitation, 72,* 127–131.

Wilms, W. (1984). Vocational education and job success: The employer's view. *Phi Delta Kappa, 65,* 347–350.

Wilson, B. (1987). Single case experimental designs in neuropsychological rehabilitation. *Journal of Clinical and Experimental Neuropsychology, 9,* 527–544.

Wilson, B. (1989). Models of cognitive rehabilitation. In R. L. Wood & P. Eames (Eds.), *Models of brain injury rehabilitation* (pp. 117–141). London: Chapman & Hall.

Wilson, B. (1992). Recovery and compensatory strategies in head injured memory impaired people several years after insult. *Journal of Neurology, Neurosurgery and Psychiatry, 55,* 177–180.

Wilson, B., & Moffat, N. (1984). Running a memory group. In B. Wilson & N. Moffat (Eds.), *Clinical management of memory problems* (pp. 171–198). London: Croom Helm.

Wolpe, J. (1961). The systematic desensitization treatment of neurosis. *Journal of Nervous and Mental Disease, 132,* 189–203.

Wolpe, J., & Lazarus, A. A. (1966). *Behavior therapy techniques: A guide to the treatment of neuroses.* Oxford: Pergamon Press.

Wood, R. L. (1984). Behavior disorders following severe brain injury: Their presentation and psychological management. In N. Brooks (Ed.), *Closed head injury: Psychological, social, and family consequences* (pp. 195–219). Oxford: Oxford University Press.

Wood, R. L. (1987). *Brain injury rehabilitation: A neurobehavioral approach.* London: Croom Helm.

Wood, R. L. (1988a). Attention disorders in brain injury rehabilitation. *Journal of Learning Disabilities, 21,* 327–332.

Wood, R. L. (1988b). Management of behavior disorders in a day treatment setting. *Journal of Head Trauma Rehabilitation, 3,* 53–61.

Wood, R. L., & Burgess, P. W. (1988). The psychological management of behavior disorders following brain injury. In I. Fussey & G. M. Giles (Eds.), *Rehabilitation of the severely brain injured adult: A practical approach* (pp. 43–68). London: Croom Helm.

Wood, R. L., & Fussey, I. (1987). Computer-based cognitive retraining: A controlled study. *International Disability Studies, 9,* 149–153.

Wroblewski, B. A., Guidos, A., Leary, J., & Joseph, A. (1992). Control of depression with fluoxetine and antiseizure medication in a brain injured patient. *American Journal of Psychiatry, 149,* 118–122.

Wroblewski, B. A., & Joseph, A. B. (1992). The use of intramuscular midazolam for acute seizure cessation or behavioral emergencies in patients with traumatic brain injury. *Clinical Neuropharmacology, 1,* 44–49.

Ylvisaker, M., & Szekeres, S. F. (1989). Metacognitive and executive impairments in head injured children and adults. *Topics in Language Disorders, 9,* 34–49.

Youngjohn, J. R., & Altman, I. M. (1989). A performance-based group approach to the treatment of anosognosia and denial. *Rehabilitation Psychology, 34,* 217–222.

Yudofsky, S., Williams, D., & Gorman, J. (1981). Propranolol in the treatment of rage and violent behavior in patients with chronic brain syndromes. *American Journal of Psychiatry, 138,* 218–220.

Zahara, D. J., & Cuvo, A. J. (1984). Behavioral applications to the rehabilitation of traumatically head injured persons. *Clinical Psychology Review, 4,* 477–491.

Zangwill, O. L. (1947). Psychological aspects of rehabilitation in cases of brain injury. *British Journal of Psychiatry, 37,* 60–69.

Zanobio, M. E. (1987). Representative neuropsychological rehabilitation programs: Italy. In M. J. Meier, A. L. Benton, & L. Diller (Eds.), *Neuropsychological rehabilitation* (pp. 406–409). New York: Churchill Livingstone.

Zeigler, E. A. (1987). Spouses of persons who are brain injured: Overlooked victims. *Journal of Rehabilitation*, January, 50–53.

Zencius, A. H., Wesolowski, M. D., Burke, W. H., & McQuade, P. (1989). Antecedent control in the treatment of brain injured clients. *Brain Injury, 3,* 199–205.

Zencius, A., Wesolowski, M. D., Krankowski, T., & Burke, W. H. (1991). Memory notebook training with traumatically brain injured clients. *Brain Injury, 5,* 321–325.

Zung, W. W. (1965). A self rating depression scale. *Archives of General Psychiatry, 12,* 63–70.

Index

MIX
Papier aus verantwortungsvollen Quellen
Paper from responsible sources
FSC® C105338

If you have any concerns about our products,
you can contact us on
ProductSafety@springernature.com

In case Publisher is established outside the EU,
the EU authorized representative is:
Springer Nature Customer Service Center GmbH
Europaplatz 3, 69115 Heidelberg, Germany

Printed by Libri Plureos GmbH
in Hamburg, Germany